PROTOCOLS FOR ELECTIVE USE
OF LIFE-SUSTAINING TREATMENTS
A Design Guide

Steven H. Miles, M.D., is an Assistant Professor of Medicine at the Pritzker School of Medicine at the University of Chicago where he is the Associate Director of the Center for Clinical Medical Ethics.

Carlos F. Gomez is a Ph.D. candidate at the Graduate School of Public Policy Studies at the University of Chicago. He is currently on academic leave from the University of Virginia School of Medicine. Mr. Gomez is a fellow in the Pew Program in Medicine, Arts, and the Social Sciences at the University of Chicago.

Christine K. Cassel, M.D., is an Associate Professor of Medicine, Chief of the Section of General Internal Medicine, and Assistant Director of the Center for Clinical Medical Ethics at the Pritzker School of Medicine at the University of Chicago.

PROTOCOLS FOR ELECTIVE USE OF LIFE-SUSTAINING TREATMENTS

A Design Guide

Steven H. Miles, M.D.
Carlos F. Gomez

Foreword by
Christine K. Cassel, M.D.

SPRINGER SCIENCE+BUSINESS MEDIA, LLC

89   90   91   92   93   /   5   4   3   2   1

ISBN 978-3-662-38660-6   ISBN 978-3-662-39522-6 (eBook)
DOI 10.1007/978-3-662-39522-6

Dedicated to
Joline
Mimi
Erica

Contents

Discusses the historical development and prevalence of hospital, nursing home, and emergency medical system protocols. The roles of professional associations, the Joint Commission, the Federal Government, and certifying bodies in promoting these protocols is examined.

Discusses the objectives of health care facility protocols in relation to the responsibilities of health care facilities, clinical decision making, and treatment-plan implementation. Reviews research on the effect of protocols on clinical care.

health care personnel and coordinating elective medical
treatment with other facilities. Discusses protocol provisions for implementing the protocol itself.

Acknowledgments

An initial draft of this book was developed under contract for the United States Congress' Office of Technology Assessment (OTA). The initial draft was adapted by OTA to its format and published in 1988 under the title, *Institutional Protocols for Decisions about Life Sustaining Treatments*. We are grateful for the assistance of Claire Maklan, Gretchen S. Kolsrud, Katy Maslow, and other OTA staff.

Early drafts of this report were critiqued by a panel of consultants that was convened by the OTA. These consultants included Marshall B. Kapp of Wright State University, C. Ross Anthony of the Health Care Financing Administration, Robert Arnold of the University of Pennsylvania School of Medicine, Mila A. Aroskar of the University of Minnesota, David Axelrod of the New York State Department of Health, Diana Bader of the Catholic Health Association, John H. Burkhart of the American Medical Association, Nancy M. Coleman of the American Bar Association, Charles J. Fahey of Fordham University, Susan Harris of the American Health Care Association, Elma Holder of the National Citizens Coalition on Nursing Home Reform, Jane Hoyt of the Nursing Home Action Group, Alan Meisel of the School of Law at the University of Pittsburgh, Nicholas Rango of the Village Nursing Home, Dorothy Rasinski-Gregory of the Veterans Administration, William A. Read of the American Hospital Association, Paul M. Schyve of the Joint Commission on Accreditation of Health Care Organizations, Alan J. Weisbard of the New Jersey Commission on Legal and Ethical Problems in the Delivery of Health Care, Susan

M. Wolf of the Hastings Center, and Stuart Youngner of the University Hospitals in Cleveland. The incisive and sometimes critical comments of these consultants make this a better work.

We are also grateful for the assistance of Dr. Christine Cassel and Dr. Mark Siegler for their critical review of this work throughout its progress. Bryan Marsh was helpful with a preliminary draft of the section on the known effects of health care facility protocols.

Dr. Miles is generously supported by the Henry J. Kaiser Family Foundation, which has named him a Faculty Scholar in General Internal Medicine.

The opinions expressed in this book are those of the authors and may not be shared by the consultants or institutions whose help we acknowledge.

Introduction

Christine K. Cassel

This book flags the development of an important aspect of biomedical ethics, the institutional and societal matrix of the elective use of life-sustaining treatments. It confirms an explicit balancing of a health care ethic heretofore centered on the physician–patient relationship with a more complex public and social ethic that acknowledges the institutional and multidisciplinary basis of modern health care. To acknowledge the need for this balance is not to relinquish the centrality of clinical care to medicine, or the moral and therapeutic importance of the clinician–patient relationship. It is, instead, to recognize the increasingly complex and public setting of the therapeutic relationship, and to establish standards for decision making and communication that will sustain and protect those relationships.

During the mid-1970s it would have been unusual for any hospital or nursing home to have a written protocol addressing decisions about the elective use of life-sustaining treatment. In California, Massachusetts, and a few other places in the mid-1970s, some hospitals were beginning to encourage physicians to actually write "Do Not Resuscitate" orders in the chart. The Beth Israel Hospital in Boston published explicit policies for decisions to forego cardiopulmonary resuscitation. The Massachusetts General Hospital described its "Optimal Care Committee" and the system of patient care categories it had instituted. These were radical moves at the time, and occasioned controversy and resistance in some hospitals. There were many reasons for controversy.

First, physicians and nurses had not considered the need or role for such explicit guides to decision making and clinical communication. To accept, even welcome, written and public protocols for the elective use of life-sustaining treatment is in some profound and public way to accept the inevitability of death as a part of clinical management. There is now an enormous literature about health care professionals' difficulties in dealing with death. Physicians in particular have been characterized as unable or unwilling to accept their own limitations, to accept human mortality, and to move gracefully from a heroic "curing" mode to a palliative "caring" mode. Clinicians often experienced a patient's death as a failure, and decisions to forgo life-sustaining treatment as somehow embarrassing, private, or as evidence of inadequacy. Life-sustaining technologies, such as ventilators and renal dialysis, once started were rarely discontinued. Medical training was notably lacking in discussions of death, of the care of the dying patient, and in developing the communication skills necessary to address such emotion-laden realities with patients and their families.

Second, professionals and lay people alike were just beginning to develop a common language for discussing these difficult confrontations with mortality within the context of rising expectations for medical miracles. The language of patient autonomy and respect for persons was just emerging from the new field of biomedical ethics. The first legal precedents for withdrawing care were being established. The Karen Ann Quinlan decision of the New Jersey Supreme Court in 1976 asserted a patient's right to refuse potentially life-sustaining treatment and recommended new institutional structures ("prognosis committees") to assist in and to validate such decisions. Many more such cases have subsequently emerged to clarify the legal framework within which these decisions can be made. The public consensus, however, is more than a merely legal framework; it encompasses the attitudes and discourse of people as experienced in their own lives and as expressed in the press, electronic media, and the culture of our society. When physicians now discuss resuscitation decisions with patients and their families, the need for and terms used in these discussions are more readily accepted and understood by all parties.

Third, hospitals, and to some degree other health care institutions, were increasingly seen as independent agents in the provision of health care. As described by Paul Starr in The Social Transformation of American Medicine (1982), prior to 1970 hospitals were simply the workplace of physicians, who had enormous, unencumbered autonomy in their decision making regarding patient care. A hospital's mission was to facilitate independent professional decision making by physicians. Hospital directors were often physicians themselves who presided over a resplendent growth in new medical technology with relatively few financial constraints. As Starr describes, in responding to new financial incentives and limits, hospitals have become an increasingly corporate culture run by professional managers with their own agendas for financial stability and growth. The independence of hospitals is importantly limited by the growth of regulation and consumer accountability. This expanded public accountability of health care administrators has resulted in more carefully articulated institutional policy positions, including policies addressing the elective use of life-sustaining treatment.

The growth of the corporate hospital was concurrent with the loss of physician autonomy in relation to the institution in the provision of health care. Hospitals are now more likely to be run by nonphysician health care administrators. The physician is more likely to be a salaried employee of a health care corporation that runs the hospital(s) or the nursing home(s). Under these conditions, private decisions made in the agony and intimacy of the doctor–patient relationship are simply inadequate to the complexity of the moral and procedural world in which decisions will be made and viewed by others including quality-assurance personnel, professional standards review organizations (PSROs), reimbursement agencies, and the multiple consultants inevitably involved in the patient's care. It is indeed no longer possible for a physician, or a patient for that matter, to ignore the importance of the institution in which health care is delivered.

Many health care facilities have an explicit moral mission, articulated and affirmed by a board of trustees. In recent years, some appellate court decisions upholding a patient's right to refuse life-sustaining treatment have sharpened the conflict between patient preferences and the missions of the involved hospital or nursing home. In some cases, patients have been transferred to other facilities; in others the facility has been directed to provide the treatment over its objections. Rather than being a silent shelter for an individual physician's or patient's decisions, health care facilities are increasingly playing an active public role in decisions about the elective use of life-sustaining treatment.

Hospitals are no longer the predominant type of health care facility in this country. Hospitals actually comprise a distinct minority of inpatient beds. There are already more nursing home beds than hospital beds, a disproportion that will continue to grow. "Long-term care facilities" themselves contain a spectrum of institutions, from skilled and intermediate-care nursing homes to rehabilitation centers and hospices. Furthermore, health care has become interinstitutional—no single institution can sponsor a plan for the elective use of life-sustaining treatment and be assured that that settles it. The need to transfer patients from one facility to another for the care of acute, intermittent, or convalescent medical problems means that there must be procedures to communicate treatment plans from institution to institution and from caregiver to caregiver, even in the absence of personal relationships between the caregivers.

In a sense, health facility protocols for elective use of life-sustaining treatment reflect the practice of "stranger medicine." Not only is the patient often a stranger to the physician and the nurse, but the multiple health care professionals involved in that patient's care are likely to be strangers to one another as well. The need for a shared understanding of the extent and, equally as important, the limits of the treatment plan is essential if we are to be able to respect the patient's preferences during the provision of care in such a complex institutional network.

This book is packed with information. It discusses the prevalence of protocols, their characteristics, and current research on how these protocols have affected clinical practices in hospitals, nursing homes, and emergency medical systems. It considers how these protocols are developed and proposes formats, paradigms, and provisions for their design. Using case vignettes, it gives examples of how protocols might assist health care staff in addressing specific clinical situations. It builds on the language of important prior work, including that of the President's Commission (1982, 1983), and discusses the role of significant professional bodies (such as the Joint Commission on the Accreditation of Health Care Organizations) in promoting health facility protocols. Indeed, it is remarkable how much there is to say on this topic.

This book is primarily intended for health care facility policymakers. Broadly defined, this audience includes professional administrators, lawyers, directors of nursing, social workers, boards of directors, ethics consultants, and clinicians who are involved in designing and implementing institutional policies for the elective use of life-sustaining treatments. Thus, this book is aimed at the health professionals who are addressing quality assurance and utilization review, who are trying to respond to the new standards of the Joint Commission for the Accreditation of Health Care Organizations (1987, 1988a, b), and who are trying to meet their public responsibility to provide better patient care. I also urge that physicians, nurses, and allied health professionals who are educators read this book; it offers assistance and perspective to their endeavors as well.

It may be important to say a few words about what this book is not. This is not a textbook of basic principles of biomedical ethics. Nor is it a set of guidelines for making decisions about the elective use of life-sustaining treatment. These important areas are amply covered by essays and books in the now substantial and established field of biomedical ethics. Principles for decision making for the elective use of life-sustaining treatment are summarized in Chapter 2. Any summary of bioethical principles is inadequate to deal with the inescapable specificity of the clinical world, and I would urge the reader to seek further discussion and understanding of these principles. Concepts such as "Do no harm" and "Respect for self-determination" have prima facie validity, but often seem to conflict in the tangle of emerging realities such as unprecedented technologies, modern information systems, and changing expectations of professional and patient alike.

Medical ethics is evolving, and scrutiny of new aspects of ethical principles will continue. For example, the acceptability of allowing a patient to die by withholding or withdrawing food and nutrition is a topic that was barely mentioned in the early 1980s. Now it has been subjected to extraordinary scrutiny and controversy in the courts as well as in the medical and legal literature. Similar discussions, such as those regarding assisted suicide and the rights and obligations of individual health care professionals and facilities, will continue in the literature. Health facility policymakers should stay informed, participate in that debate, and will find it helpful to refer to the appended bibliography of texts and periodicals for additional information not covered herein.

Protocols are not ethical principles or moral dictates. Although they are based in the shared moral assumptions of a pluralistic society, they rarely include specific moral proscriptions, for example, against physician-assisted suicide. The notion of protocols described in this book encompasses two aspects of clinical practice: decision making and treatment-plan implementation. Protocols are most readily recognized as guidelines for decision making in the "public" forum of health care institutions. Institutions should consider how to encourage deeper discussion of the moral principles underlying clinical decisions so as to allow a full and meaningful examination of dilemmas that will be difficult regardless of how well the protocol is designed. These kinds of discussions can be promoted through a combination of in-service training, ethics committees, or study-group discussions (see Chapter 4).

Health care facility protocols reflect that health care is no longer practiced in an entirely unquestioned private encounter with patients. Public policies for the protection of patients' rights, to ensure quality of care, or to control the appropriateness of reimbursement may threaten privacy. But, if clinicians understand the genesis of policies and regulations, they need not forego personal involvement with patients, compassion and empathy, respect for the dignity of life, and pathos at its tragedies. Clinicians should not allow their frustration with the limits and rigidities of health care bureaucracies to interfere with our work and care. All of the richness that is involved in the care of the sick remains if we know how to seek it and advocate for it.

This book promotes a vital view of health facility protocols. At their best, institutional protocols affirm that private space and discretion is still essential to the care of the sick. Protocols give permission; it is not necessary to go through courts, lawsuits, or endless committees to provide good health care. Protocols should encourage accountable health care professionals through shared and advance decision making with autonomous patients to create a private space where the curtains can be safely drawn and intensely personal decisions made by those most intimately involved.

PART I
Current Protocol Practices and Objectives

CHAPTER 1
The Evolution of Health Care Facility Protocols

The view that life-sustaining treatments are *elective* is a profound challenge to patients, the medical profession, and to health care facilities. For patients, the term *elective* is a query that requires an answering commitment to pursue or decline this treatment, at this time, in these circumstances. For health care professionals, elective implies something quite unlike the view that treatment decisions are about medical "indications," a language that speaks of technical duties that follow a professional discernment. For a health care facility with a mission to respect life, an elective view of treatment transforms the presumption in favor of treatment into an interim safeguard to be ratified by an individual choice so that patient care serves personal needs, not public rhetoric.

The elective use of life-sustaining treatments encompasses the choice to pursue, to decline, or to withdraw from therapies. Much has been made of a patient's right to forego overtreatment. There is also a right to choose therapy, to avoid the undertreatment that is possible when the disabled and chronically ill are stigmatized and not listened to. The need for collaborative, comprehensive treatment planning is implicit in the elective use of life-sustaining treatments. The physician's expertise, experience, and judgment is part of a partnership of shared decision making with patients who elect how to live with their illnesses and available treatment options.

HISTORY

Health care facility protocols to improve the elective use of life-sustaining treatments have emerged at the confluence of three major changes in the American health care delivery system: (1) the development of new life-sustaining technologies, (2) changes in the role of patients in treatment decision making, and (3) an expanded view of the responsibilities of health care facilities. Although these changes set the stage for health care facility protocols, the impetus for protocols came from a perception that physicians or health care facilities were unwilling to allow patients' views or interests to guide decisively the use of life-sustaining treatments. Thus, the years since the late 1970s have borne witness to court decisions, laws (e.g., living wills), and health care facility protocols that affirm that life-sustaining treatments are elective and that patients must have the decisive role in guiding their use. A familiarity with the history of these *protocols* (a term we use in order to include policies as well as guidelines) is useful to understanding why these protocols exist in their current format and why they continue to be so problematic.

The simultaneous introduction of defibrillation, mouth-to-mouth ventilation, and external cardiac massage in the late 1950s transformed the hospital management of sudden death. Cardiac-arrest teams, mobile carts for resuscitation equipment, coronary care units, and nurses trained in defibrillation techniques quickly followed in the early and middle 1960s (President's Commission, 1983). The medical community immediately recognized that cardiopulmonary resuscitation (CPR), which was developed as a therapy for unexpected cessation of cardiorespiratory function, was a unique kind of therapy (Debard, 1981; Kouwenhoven, Jude, & Knickerbocker, 1960). Beginning in 1962 and continuing to the present, an unprecedented series of National Conference consensus statements from the American Heart Association, the National Academy of Science, the American Red Cross, and other prestigious groups, has set standards for the use of this technology. These statements have mirrored changes in the public policy view of medical ethics.

The unique urgency of the treatment of cardiac arrest led the National Conference to propose that health personnel initiate CPR without waiting for a formal order from the attending physician (1974). The presumption in favor of initiating CPR without a physician's written order nevertheless assumed that this new technology would be used judiciously. As the 1974 consensus paper put it, "the physician has an obligation to initiate CPR in any situation where it is medically indicated," noting that the absence of medical indications "such as terminal irreversible illness where death is not unexpected" would lead the judicious physician to see that CPR was not given (National Conference, 1974, p. 834). This view of "medically indicated CPR" did not refer to patient preferences. Because of the impossibility of determining whether CPR was indicated at the time of an arrest, the 1974 Commission recommended that the physician note an order to withhold resuscitation in the patient's progress notes and on the physician's order sheet. The first hospital CPR protocols soon followed (Executive Committee, 1976; Longo, Warren, & Roberts, 1988; Miles & Moldow, 1984).

The landmark Quinlan decision by the New Jersey Supreme Court in 1976 emphasized the role of the patient's views in decisions about life-sustaining medical treatments. This legal development was based on legal support for a person's right to be free from unconsented invasions and from the need for informed consent as a prerequisite to medical treatment (Katz, 1984). This view has been extended through a number of court decisions (Doudera, 1982), a prestigious President's Commission (President's Commission, 1982, 1983), and statements by medical and nonmedical bodies (e.g., American College of Physicians, 1986; Concern for Dying, 1987; Hastings Center, 1987; New York State, 1987).

This strong emphasis on patient preferences in health care decisions has settled uneasily into the medical profession's view of decision making that has been centered on medical indications (Katz, 1984). Although physicians are now more likely to inform patients of life threatening diseases, they still inadequately apprise patients of treatment options and often do not involve them in critical decisions about life-sustaining treatments (Bedell, 1986; Bedell & Delbanco, 1984; President's Commission, 1982). The language of medical indications still echoes in legal opinions (*In re Dinnerstein*, 1978), and in articles on medical ethics that propose that the physician need not offer or provide futile life-sustaining care (Blackhall, 1987; Hastings Center, 1987; Steinbrook & Lo, 1988). This ambivalence was again reflected in the 1980 CPR consensus statement (American Heart Association, 1980). The vague and probabilistic nature of futility and the fear of misused medical paternalism has relegated a medical-indications view of decisions about life-sustaining care to the background. A 1987 government report suggested that futility had virtually no role in treatment decisions because medical certainty is rarely obtainable (Office of Technology Assessment, 1987), a proposition that no doubt strikes many lay persons and professionals confronting end-stage degenerative diseases as unhelpful. The difficulty balancing the relative roles of medical expertise and patient preferences in health care decisions has been a powerful impetus for health care facility policies and guidelines. They are designed to promote a decision-making process where the patient's experience and preferences are decisive factors in the construction of a treatment plan for the use of life-sustaining treatments.

A profound expansion in the public view of the responsibilities of health care institutions, occurring concurrently with changes in life-sustaining technologies and medical decision making, was the final social change that led to health care facility protocols for the elective use of life-sustaining treatment. Before this change, treatment decisions were a matter of an independent physician's medical judgment, rather than an institutional concern; hospital protocols that proposed otherwise would have been considered an unwarranted intrusion on medical practice. These institutional responsibilities are examined in Chapter 2.

In 1976—the year of the *Quinlan* decision—the *New England Journal of Medicine* published two hospital protocols addressing decisions about life-sustaining treatments (Clinical Care Committee, 1976; Rabkin, Gillerman, & Rice, 1976), with an enthusiastic editorial entitled "Terminating Life Support: Out of the Closet!" (Fried, 1976). These protocols were by no means the first,* but their assertive presentation in a prestigious medical journal marked a new phase in the use of health care facility protocols to reconcile powerful medical technologies with a new view of medical decision making and institutional responsibility.

These forces have had a profound impact on medical practice. In that nearly all do-not-resuscitate (DNR) orders are accompanied by decisions to withhold a cluster of life-sustaining treatments, the prevalence of DNR orders reflects the prevalence of decisions to withhold other life-sustaining therapies. DNR orders are currently written on 4% to 13% of all hospitalized patients (Evans & Brody, 1985; Lo, Seika, Strulla, Thomas, & Showstock; 1985; Schwartz & Reilly, 1986) Such orders precede 70% to 75% of all deaths on general wards (Bedell et al., 1986; Levy, Lambe, & Shear, 1984) and 30% to 40% of deaths of intensive care patients (Witte, 1984; Zimmerman et al., 1986). One-fifth of dialysis patients died from elective withdrawal of dialysis (Neu & Kjellstrand, 1986), a figure that may be doubled in elderly dialysis patients (Office of Technology Assessment [OTA], 1987) Antibiotics may be electively withheld from 20% to 40% of nursing home patients (Brown & Thompson, 1979; Office of Technology Assessment, 1987). One-half of nursing home patients in one study had some limitation on the use of life-sustaining therapies (Mott & Barker, 1988).

HOSPITALS

Hospitals have developed protocols at an increasing pace since the 1976 Quinlan decision (see Figure 1.1 and Table 1.1). Recent surveys find that 35% to 70% of hospitals have protocols, mainly do-not-resuscitate (DNR)

---

* Institutional hospice models for palliative care of dying patients date to the early 1950s (Saunders, 1977).

protocols, addressing decisions about life-sustaining treatment (Hospital Council, 1984; Miles & Moldow, 1984; Mozdzierz & Schlesinger, 1986; New York State Task Force, 1987; Office of Technology Assessment, 1987). These protocols are most common in larger hospitals and in those with academic or church affiliations. They are present in a large majority of hospitals with more than 200 beds; most hospitals without protocols are very small, rural facilities. Little is known about the presumably great state-to-state variation in the prevalence or design of protocols in response to variations in state law or local leadership.

Typically, hospital protocols address acute care and intensive care issues such as DNR orders, though more recently developed protocols address a broader range of life-sustaining treatments (Figure 1.1). The recent evolution of hospital protocols beyond the narrow scope of intensive life support reflects an expanding consensus that the moral and legal principles developed for the DNR decision apply to decision making for all life-sustaining

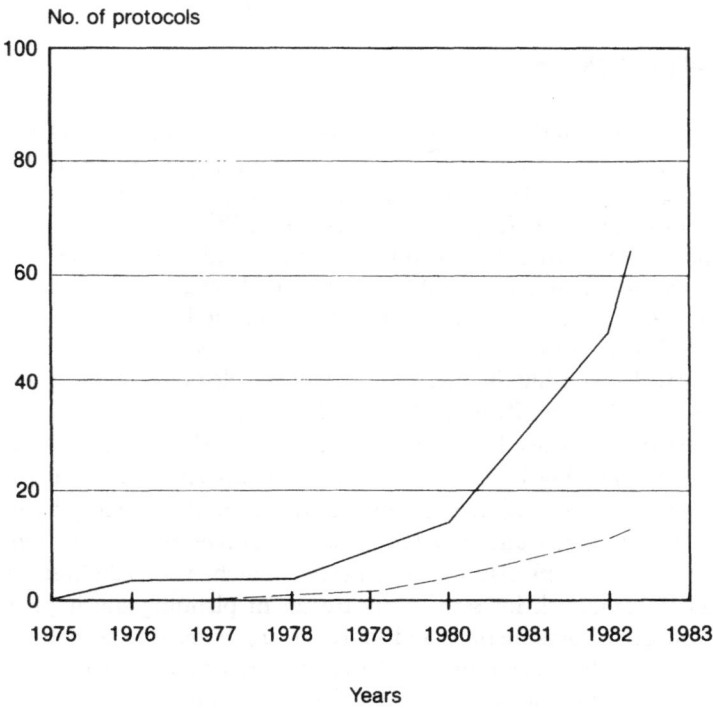

FIGURE 1.1 Cumulative adoption of hospital protocols for limiting treatment. *Solid line:* DNR; *dashed line:* Supportive care only.

From Miles and Moldow, 1984.

therapies. A New York State Task Force study (1987) has found that many of these protocols now address the determination of decision-making capacity as well, content that was not a prominent feature of protocols before the 1982 President's Commission discussion of decision-making capacity (President's Commission, 1982; Miles & Moldow, 1984).

Many hospital protocols have been published (Arena, Perlin, & Turnbull, 1980; Beth Israel, 1982; City of Boston, 1983; Committee on Policy, 1983; Clinical Care, 1976; Davila, Boisaubin, & Sears, 1986; Duff, 1979; Executive Committee, 1976; Halligan & Hamel, 1985; Los Angeles, 1983; McPhail, Moore, O'Connor, & Woodward, 1981; Meisel, Grenvil, Pinkus, & Snyder, 1986; Miles, Cranford, & Schultz, 1982; Mount Sinai Hospital, 1984; Northwestern Memorial Hospital, 1982; Quill, Stankiti, & Kraus, 1986; Somerville Hospital, 1983; St. Joseph's, 1984a; St. Joseph's, 1984b; St. Joseph's, 1984c; St. Joseph's, 1984d; St. Joseph's, 1984e; University of Wisconsin, 1983; Van Eys, Bowen, & Alt, 1986; Volicer, 1986). (See Appendix I for selected sample protocols.)

NURSING HOMES

Long-term care facilities are following the lead of hospitals after a lag of 3 to 4 years. (See Table 1.1.) About 20% to 35% of nursing homes have adopted written policies for decisions about life-sustaining treatment (Miles & Ryden, 1985; Office of Technology Assessment, 1987). One study's surprisingly high finding that 41% of nursing homes had a policy was probably skewed by the urban nature of their sample and because the researchers did not confirm that written protocols actually existed (Levinson, Shepard, Dunn, & Parker, 1987). Glasser's finding that 61% of homes have protocols probably reflects an highly unrepresentative sample of facilities due to a low response rate (Glasser, Zweibel, & Cassel, 1988).

A variety of forces have contributed to the slower development of protocols for nursing homes. Most published models have been designed for hospitals and do not address nursing home needs. Nursing homes are smaller than hospitals and may have fewer resources available for protocol drafting. Smaller staffs also may not need as much of an administrative or procedural framework for satisfactory treatment planning and implementation. Professional organizations and some nursing home operators have been reluctant to codify decision-making procedures. Responses to a recent survey of 75 nursing homes as to why they did not have protocols included statements that the idea of protocols had not occurred to the administrators or that they felt that protocols were unnecessary. These administrators also said that the absence of protocols allowed for administrative simplicity and flexibility,

TABLE 1.1   Prevalence of Protocols for Elective Use of Life-Sustaining Treatments

	1976	1977	1978	1979	1980	1981	1982	1983	1984	1985	1986
						% with policies					
						Hospitals					
Miles	2	3	3	7	14	35	42	46			
Longo											57
Mozdierz							35				
						Nursing Homes					
Longo*											20
Miles							4		16		
Levinson									41		

*Includes formal protocols only.
Statistics are from Longo, 1988; Miles & Moldow, 1984; Levinson, et al., 1987.

avoided legal exposure, did not intrude on the physician–patient relationship, and that practices in this area were well known anyway (Glasser et al., 1988).

Typical nursing home protocols address a broader range of treatment issues than do hospital protocols (Miles, Gomez, Cassel, & Zweibel, 1988). Protocols for categories of care address CPR, feeding, antibiotics, and transfer to acute care facilities (Besdine, 1983; Brown & Thompson, 1979; Greenlaw, 1982; Hilfiker, 1983; Levenson, 1981; Miles & Ryden, 1985; Mott & Barker, 1988; Yarows, 1987). Reflecting the greater prominence of nursing and social work staff in managing patient care, these protocols often describe more extensive duties for intake social workers and primary care nurses than do hospital protocols (Levinson et al., 1987, Miles & Ryden, 1985). Many of these protocols may be deficient in their normative description of a good decision-making process, and may omit provisions for resident autonomy or documentation (Miles & Ryden, 1985). To the extent that these deficiencies reflect clinical practices, they strongly argue for improved training of nursing home staff and administrators in the elective use of life-sustaining treatment.

A few nursing home protocols or models have been published (Ad hoc Committee, 1985; Hoyt & Davies, 1984, 1986; Levenson, List, & Zaw-Win, 1981; Mott & Barker, 1988; Task Force, 1984; Uhlmann, Cassel, & McDonald, 1987; Yarows, 1987).

EMERGENCY MEDICAL SYSTEMS

A few emergency medical systems (EMS) have developed protocols that allow paramedics or hospital emergency rooms to accept DNR orders from nursing homes or hospice home care programs. Some protocols have been integrated into ambulance service protocols (Marshall, 1985; Miles & Crimmins, 1985; Minnesota Medical Association Trustees, 1986). One policy was implemented by a small group practice working with a single hospital and a single nursing home (Mott & Barker, 1988) Such protocols or understandings are essential if nursing home or home care patients are to be able to decline CPR or other life-sustaining treatments in a health care system that often transfers patients between health care facilities just as urgent medical indications for such treatments arise (Haynes & Niemann, 1985; Miles, 1987).

To be fully effective in a multiple-provider system, hospital protocols have to allow emergency admission staff to accept directives that have been given to EMS providers from nursing home, home care agency records, or properly identified surrogates. One symposium extensively discusses the tragic overtreatment that can occur with the presently inadequate emergency-admission policies for receiving advance directives (Death at a New York Hospital, 1985).

The integration of policy and practice for interfacility transfers can be quite complex (Besdine, 1983; Hilfiker, 1983; Levenson et al., 1981). Without these policies, some nursing home staff, aware of EMS standing orders for CPR, choose not to summon EMS care for patients who have declined CPR. This practice can deprive such persons of other, desired life-sustaining or palliative treatments for distressful or life-threatening conditions, such as pulmonary edema. With clear interfacility understandings, excellent control of patient care can be obtained without restricting access to a desired level of emergency care (Mott & Barker, 1988).

Special procedural principals for EMS system protocols have been proposed (Miles & Crimmins, 1985). Coordinated protocols between EMS providers, nursing homes, and hospitals must standardize the terminology to be used in such orders. Procedures for rapidly verifying the proper authority of the directive need to be created. The facility that gives the original orders must be willing to take full responsibility for the decision-making process that created the order. To accomplish this coordination, the Minneapolis EMS system proposed model nursing home and home care policies to go with the protocols that were enacted within the EMS system proper (Miles & Crimmins, 1985; Minnesota Medical, 1986). The EMS system in a small city maintained a list of patients with DNR orders who might be receiving medical care (Marshall, 1985). To be fully effective, emergency hospital admission policies will have to provide for the acceptance of directives that have been given to EMS providers from nursing home or home care agency records.

The American College of Emergency Physicians has resolved to develop a model policy to address do-not-resuscitate orders by emergency medical systems (American College of Emergency Physicians, 1985, Board of Directors, 1986, 1987). Protocols that provide for advance planning, written accountability for treatment decisions, and clear communications will be necessary to ensure patient autonomy in a multifacility health care system where interim providers are completely unfamiliar with the history of patients they treat.

PROFESSIONAL BODIES AND CERTIFYING BOARDS

Numerous professional associations have proposed decision-making approaches for life-sustaining treatment. The role of the consensus guidelines on CPR was mentioned above (National Conference, 1986). The American Medical Association has framed such decisions from a standpoint of patient' rights and consent (American Medical Association, 1986). By 1985, 40% of state medical associations had adopted model protocols or model guidelines (unpublished data by R. Anderson & S.H. Miles). The American Hospital Association has issued a patient bill of rights (American Hospital Association, 1973, 1985) and has emphasized the assurance of quality patient care—including termination-of-treatment decisions—as the overriding responsibility of all health care facilities (American Hospital Association, 1985). Sixty percent of state hospital associations (Office of Technology Assessment, 1987), the Veterans Administration (1984), the American College of Emergency Physicians (1985), the American Health Care Association (1981), National Institutes of Health (1983), city health departments (Bar Association, 1983), ad hoc groups (Task Force, 1984; Uhlmann et al., 1987) and other bodies have also developed models.

The Joint Commission on Accreditation of Health Care Organizations has become increasingly involved in setting protocol standards for the elective use of life-sustaining treatments. In addition to mandating minimum standards for the technical provision of such treatments, the Joint Commission has recently required accredited acute-care and long-term care facilities to develop and implement protocols that specifically address decisions to withhold resuscitation (see Appendix III). Joint Commission standards for hospitals and nursing homes now require that the chief executive officer consult with medical and nursing staffs and other "appropriate" consultants to develop a policy that:

1. Defines procedures for the resolution of conflicts in this area
2. Assures that patients' rights are respected

3. States that DNR orders may be written *only* by the physician primarily responsible for the patient
4. Requires complete documentation of DNR orders in the patient's chart.

Similar standards have been enacted for Joint Commission accredited psychiatric, rehabilitation, and drug-dependency facilities (Joint Commission, 1987). Moreover, standards for accredited nursing homes and other long-term care facilities have been enacted since April of 1988. These new standards require that the governing body of the hospital give formal approval before the policy becomes effective (Joint Commission, 1988).

These new Joint Commission standards may be expected to have a profound impact on the development of DNR policies. The Joint Commission accredits more than 5,000 of the 6,000 general hospitals in this country, and over 3,000 other health care facilities. At present, slightly fewer than 10% of the 19,000 long-term care facilities in this country are accredited by the Joint Commission. Nevertheless, the stature of the Joint Commission means that even non-accredited health care facilities will have an incentive to develop comparable DNR protocols because Joint Commission standards may be used to evaluate the practices at any health care facility (see Chapter 2).

The Health Care Financing Administration (HCFA), which indirectly regulates the quality of a large number of acute-care and long-term care facilities through its certification for Medicare reimbursement, only indirectly addresses this issue in its certification process. HCFA mandates that its certified facilities protect and promote patients' rights, provide an internal quality assurance mechanism, conform to existing state and federal practices, and provide a mechanism to address patient grievances (HCFA, 1979).

A number of nonmedical associations are also involved in the development of public policy regarding decisions about life-sustaining treatments (Grand Jury, 1985; Hastings Center, 1987; Koop and Grant, 1986). The U.S. Congress Office of Technology Assessment has addressed these protocols in two reports (Office of Technology Assessment, 1987, 1988). The National Conference of Commissioners on Uniform State Laws has issued a model *Uniform Rights of the Terminally Ill Act* to attempt to set a national legislative standard defining the rights of patients to decline life-sustaining treatments (Society for the Right To Die, 1987). The Hastings Center (1987) as well as consumer groups (Hoyt & Davies, 1986), have also addressed these issues. The Society for the Right To Die and Concern for Dying have been involved in lobbying efforts ranging from repeal of laws defining suicide as a crime, to more recent efforts to formalize the rights of patients to refuse treatment through advance directives (Concern for Dying, 1987; Koop & Grant, 1986).

SUMMARY

Recent developments in life-sustaining technologies, the emergence of strong role for patient preferences in the election of life-sustaining treatments, and changes in the governance duties of health facilities, have promoted the use of protocols to address the elective use of life-sustaining treatments. Hospitals, nursing homes, and emergency care systems have all grappled with the design and use of these protocols. The Joint Commission along with professional and governmental organizations have affirmed the conclusion that these protocols are a constructive instrument in the delivery of patient care.

CHAPTER 2

The Objectives of Health Care Facility Protocols

Health facility administrators create policies and guidelines to promote treatment practices that conform to the views and interests to which the facility is accountable. With regard to designing protocols to improve the elective use of life-sustaining treatments, attention has focused on decision making (e.g., affirmations of patient autonomy or the need for advance treatment planning) and treatment implementation (e.g., interstaff communication). Less attention has been paid to how the elective use of life-sustaining treatments affects the totality of responsibilities of health care facilities. In this broader setting, these administrative protocols not only advance a new view of patient-centered decision making, but also mediate a diverse and to some degree conflicting set of institutional duties.

The effects of failing to appreciate the mediating role of these protocols may be seen in several ways. Some nursing homes, responding to the consensus that life-sustaining treatment can be withheld, have adopted protocols that do not take account of public concern that treatment decisions be made from the patient's perspective (Miles & Ryden, 1985). The removal of procedural barriers to physician–patient decision making may have dismantled procedural safeguards that were created to protect the interests of vulnerable patients (Hoyt & Davies, 1986; Koop & Grant, 1986). Patient autonomy has not been reconciled with the fact that some health care facilities affirm health care missions that, in some cases, may fundamentally conflict with some patients' preferences. This chapter considers the design and objectives of protocols for the elective use of life-sustaining treatment in relation to the total governance agenda of health care facilities.

INSTITUTIONS AND PUBLIC INTERESTS

Health care facilities are accountable to a variety of public and private interests (see Figure 2.1). This accountability is to patients, to legal views of the public good, to moral communities (as with sectarian facilities), and to standards of good medical care. This accountability is enforced through civil liabilities, legally mandated procedures, accrediting requirements, and by voluntary compliance with a mission statement. A health care facility's board is responsible for governing the facility in a manner that advances these interests. This complex set of accountabilities is the substance of "institutional conscience" to which patients and families, staff, administrators, the public, and relevant

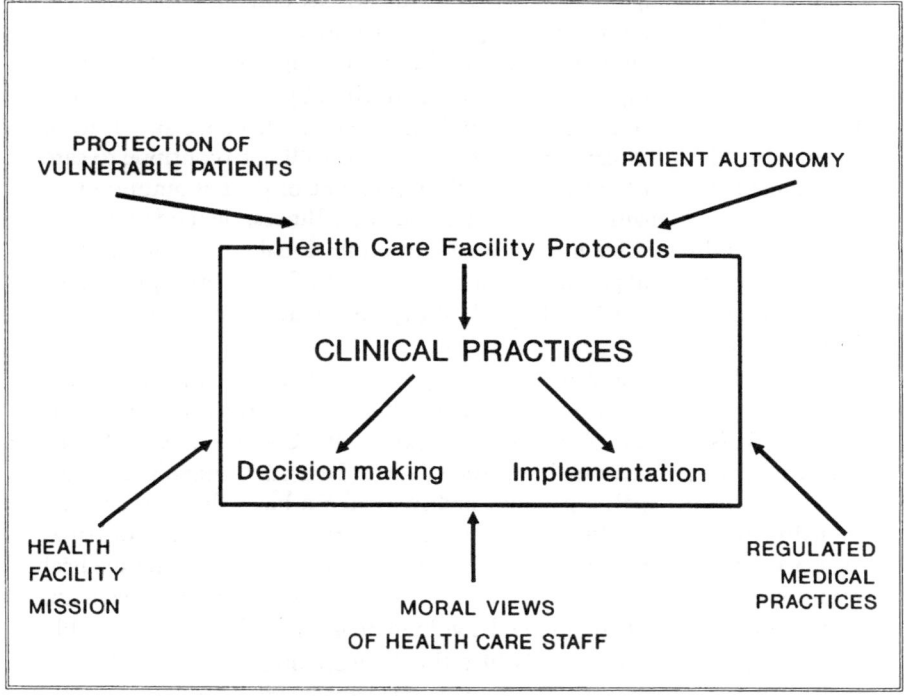

FIGURE 2.1 The setting of health care facility protocols.

moral communities may hold the facility. Chapter 6 discusses how a protocol might articulate these interests.

Five interests are especially relevant to protocols addressing the elective use of life-sustaining treatment (Figure 2.1). First, health care facilities are responsible for protecting the patient's right to exercise autonomy over his or her health care decisions. Patient autonomy is supported in statutory law, constitutional law, and in case law, as well as in a bioethical consensus (Annas, 1982; Hastings Center, 1987; Katz, 1984; Office of Technology Assessment, 1987; President's Commission, 1983). Bills of patients' rights and health professional groups have affirmed the importance of this interest to health care facilities (e.g., American Health Care Association, 1981; American Hospital Association, 1973; American Medical Association, 1986; Joint Commission, 1987).

Though patient autonomy is usually considered to be a decisive private interest in decisions about the elective use of life-sustaining treatment, treatment choices are to some degree public acts, which thus may be properly constrained by public policy (Takken, 1987). Patient autonomy has been an insufficient claim to support a request to receive a lethal injection. Even within the range of legally permitted actions, patient autonomy may be procedurally encumbered, though not abrogated, to advance other public interests. Thus, though a patient may have a right to withdraw from feeding, the competing rights of a physician who objects to this choice may mean that the patient may have to undergo the inconvenience and delay of transferring his or her care to a physician who is willing to continue to care for the patient in that manner. Finally, the extent of patient autonomy in clinical practice remains a matter of conjecture. Illness, dependency, fear, ignorance, and pervasive institutional and professional cues about desired behavior are powerful psychological constraints on the possibility of autonomy in health care settings (Cassel, 1987; Presidents Commission, 1982; Siegler, 1981).

Second, health care facilities are responsible for advancing the welfare of vulnerable persons who are unable to effectively advocate on their own behalf (Hoyt & Davies, 1986; Koop & Grant, 1986; Uddo, 1986). All health facility patients are vulnerable to some degree: Fear and unfamiliarity with the environment impair a patient's ability to act on his or her own behalf. Similarly, the failure of health professionals to perceive the needs of particular patients (e.g., an inability to speak the language or understand medical terminology or choices) can enhance patients' vulnerability (Freedman, 1978; Goodin, 1985). Patients can be vulnerable in several ways. Vulnerable persons might: (1) be so ill or disabled that they are unable to leave a facility or challenge its practices; (2) be unaware of their procedural and legal rights; (3) be without decision-making capacity or the ability to protect their own interests; (4) lack family or friends to advocate their interests should they be disabled from speaking on their own behalf; or (5) belong to classes of persons, such as the old or disabled, whose interests are endangered through social prejudices or stigmatization.

Vulnerability can affect medical decision making in several ways. The choice to not offer or withdraw life-sustaining treatment from stigmatized patients according to "substituted judgment" or a view of their "best interests," even by well-intentioned professional caregivers, can reflect social prejudices about the quality of life of disabled persons (Pearlman & Jonsen, 1985; Pearlman & Uhlmann, 1988; [Rothenbergs dissent] Hastings Center, 1987) or caregiver fatigue (Anonymous, 1988). The relentless and universal use of life-sustaining treatment can also violate a vulnerable person's dignity and right to individualized treatment planning based on their interests and views (Death at a New York Hospital, 1985).

The public interest in protecting vulnerable persons has been advanced by procedures for oversight of treatment decisions for these persons (see Chapter 8). Federal and state governments have attempted to regulate health facility practices with regard to vulnerable persons by establishing public guardians, ombudsmen, and vulnerable-adult protection acts. Several authors have pointed out that recent efforts to promote patient autonomy in decisions to withdraw life-sustaining treatments may have compromised these protections (Annas, 1984; Dornette, 1977; Hoyt & Davies, 1986, 1984; Johnson, 1985; Koop & Grant, 1986).

Third, some health care facilities are voluntarily accountable to particular health care missions (American Hospital Association, 1985; Pellegrino & Thomasma, 1981; Thomasma, 1985). Health facility mission statements advance a particular view of "good" health care in order to appeal to a particular community of patients. These missions might reflect a relationship between the facility and a moral community, as with facilities that are founded, operated, or funded by a religious community. In this case, protocols may affirm church doctrine as, for example, a Catholic hospital's policy of not performing abortions (Paris, 1987) or a Jehovah's Witness view on blood transfusions. Health care facility mission may also reflect a strategy to attract patients by means of a certain treatment philosophy (as with hospice facilities). Hospices would have a view of appropriate care of persons with advanced cancer that differs from that of a tertiary cancer-research center.

Recent court opinions have advanced a disturbing new view of health care facilities whereby each hospital or nursing home may be compelled to accede to all requests by patients, even when the request contradicts the mission of the facility (In re Bartling, 1984; In re Requenna, 1986; In re Bouvia, 1986; In re Jobes, 1987). As one ethicist-lawyer has said, "Hospitals are corporations that have no natural personhood, and hence are incapable of having either 'moral' or 'ethical objections' to actions . . . Hospitals don't practice medicine, physicians do" (Annas, 1987, p. 20). This new view would supplant a historical tradition, elaborated as recently as 1982 by The President's Commission (1982) and in 1985 by the American Hospital Association (1985) that each health care facility "has the prerogative to develop a mission reflecting its historical roots and philosophy" (p. 4). The diversity of health care facilities' missions reflects the diversity of voluntary moral communities in society. Support for these missions has presumed that patients and professionals should be able to seek and create facilities that are committed to a view of health care that is similar to their own (Emanuel, 1988; Kapp, 1987; Paris, 1987).

Fourth, health care facilities should provide for the accommodation of the moral views of their staff about patient care. As society has supported a stronger, more decisive role for patients in deciding on the elective use of life-sustaining treatments, practitioners are more likely to object to the final treatment plan. Though a physician's objections ought not to override a patient's preferences, there is a public interest in not compelling health professionals to perform duties they find morally objectionable. Our society's value on moral pluralism and voluntarism weighs against compelling providers with principled objections to participating in treatment plans (Lynn, 1987). The moral views of health care professionals are probably important means by which integrity of treatment practices and quality of care are enhanced (Brett & McCullough, 1986). The concept of "shared decision making" between patients and physicians includes the proposal that the treatment relationship be mutually voluntary and the treatment plan mutually acceptable (President's Commission, 1982, 1983). Health care facility protocols should anticipate these moral differences and provide for exempting conscientiously objecting staff from objectionable treatment plans (Hastings Center, 1987).

Fifth, health care facilities are responsible for ensuring that medical practices do not violate the law or accrediting standards. Certain treatment practices are specifically addressed; the intentional administration of lethal agents is prohibited by criminal codes. Facilities that violate these standards face possible criminal, regulatory, or civil sanctions, including fines, loss of required or prestigious accreditations, loss of operating licenses, being placed in public receivership, having admissions suspended, losing teaching programs or prestigious affiliations or accreditations (Grand Jury, 1985; Johnson, 1985; Jost, 1985). Nothing in these standards prevents a facility from allowing patients to refuse life-sustaining medical treatment (Byrne, 1982). Some facilities have inappropriately restricted a patient's right to direct their treatment because of uncertainty about the legality of withholding of life-sustaining treatment. Recent court decisions, professional statements, national commissions, and legislative actions have resolved many of these uncertainties.

Though the questions about the permissibility of withholding life-sustaining treatment have been largely addressed, new financial arrangements have raised questions about institutional interests in such decisions. Capitated reimbursement plans (e.g., federal diagnosis related groups (DRGs) reimbursements or private health maintenance organization (HMO) or preferred provider organization (PPO) capitated payment plans) operate directly on health facilities; the financial survival of a facility may depend on its ability to control costs generated by individual patient care decisions. Profit-sharing arrangements have created a similar conflict of interest for physicians who may receive a bonus if patient-care costs are contained (Everitt, 1985; Hilman, 1987; Levinson, 1987). There is concern that an ethic permitting the withholding of life-sustaining therapies presents, at least, a conflict of interest between the institution and the patient, and at worst an incentive to rationalize treatment decisions that reflect the financial interests of the health care provider. Chapter 7 addresses protocol provisions to address this issue.

CIVIL LIABILITY AND HEALTH CARE FACILITY PROTOCOLS

An older view of health care facilities as "empty shells" in which patients were treated by legally responsible professionals has been replaced by a stronger view of institutional liability to patients for treatment practices (Bertolet & Goldsmith, 1980; Kapp, 1987; Peters & Peraino, 1984). A judgment against the facility would rest on a finding that administrative action or inaction was causally connected to the injury of a patient (Curran, 1984; Southwick, 1973). The mistaken notion that written protocols for the elective use of life-sustaining treatment increase a facility's exposure to liability is slowly giving way to the view that protocols are a standard feature of good facility governance and reflect the quality of administration (Burmeister, 1986).

A health facility might be found to be *indirectly* or *vicariously* liable for an injury to a patient because of its relationship to patients through its staff. Thus, a facility might be found liable for injuries resulting from its staff's negligent performance of duties if the administration failed to provide for adequate communication between health care staff or failed to have a program to identify and address common problem areas in clinical practices (Kapp, 1987).

A facility might also be found to be *directly* liable to the patient for injuries sustained during treatment (Kapp, 1987; Peters & Peraino, 1984; Southwick, 1973). The 1965 *Darling* decision, which established the direct liability of health care facilities, allowed accrediting standards to be accepted as evidence of a standard for practice (Bertolet & Goldsmith, 1980; Peters & Peraino, 1984). Since *Darling*, the standards of state health departments or accrediting bodies have often been used to evaluate health facility negligence. Other sources of a standard for acceptable care can include statutory law, common law, constitutional principles, customary standards for medical practice, or health care facility protocols (Kapp, 1985, 1987; Peters & Peraino, 1984). Even if a facility is not required to conform to a prestigious medical association's model protocol, divergence from such a model, if causally related to a patient's injury, could be construed as negligent administration.

Legal scholars have proposed several administrative duties that may apply to protocols for the elective use of life-sustaining treatment (Bertolet & Goldsmith, 1980; Kapp, 1987; Peters & Peraino, 1984). This includes duties (1) to develop and promulgate protocols for patient care and safety; (2) to properly select, train, and supervise employees of the facility; and (3) to supervise independent contractors who provide services to patients.

Few courts have considered these duties with explicit regard to protocols for elective use of life sustaining treatments. A New York grand jury concluded that a hospital's use of colored dots on a nonpermanent record instead of medical order to withhold resuscitation "eliminated professional accountability, invited clerical error, and discouraged physicians from obtaining informed consent" (Deputy Attorney General, 1983; Grand Jury, p. 368, 1985; Youngner, 1987). A lower court in Minnesota overturned a hospital DNR order because a guardian did not understand the treatment implications of the order (*Hoyt v St. Mary's*, 1981) in a decision in which the judge cited the DNR definition of the state medical association. Other decisions have evaluated the standing of health facility missions, as was discussed earlier.

THE MEDIATING ROLE OF HEALTH CARE FACILITY PROTOCOLS

The institutional accountability of a health care facility was created to promote patients' and the public's interests. In that these interests are grounded on a vision of good health care, they usually converge with the patient's interests. A patient's interests are directly served by public support for patient autonomy and for institutional liability for health care practices. The patient's interest in quality health care is also served by the standards of accrediting or regulatory bodies. As members of sectarian communities, patients are served by the availability of health care facilities that strive to reflect the patient's own moral views in the provision of care. Vulnerable and stigmatized persons are served by the special interest in their welfare. However, the diversity of moral views among patients, providers, and within the society at large can lead to tensions within the framework for institutional accountabilities that pertain to the elective use of life sustaining treatments. This tension is especially clearly revealed in two troublesome policy-making dilemmas.

First, there is the tension between the goal of unencumbered exercise of patient autonomy and the need for procedural oversight to protect the interests of vulnerable persons. Oversight procedures for vulnerable persons should not be so cumbersome, time consuming, or costly as to prevent a competent person from directing his or her care. Thus, it is unreasonable to propose (and inaccurate to assume) that all life-sustaining treatments should be given unless court approval has been obtained to do otherwise. On the other hand, procedures to allow patients to decline life-sustaining treatments cannot be so perfunctory as to prevent procedural oversight of patients who might be improperly induced to refuse or incorrectly construed as refusing life-sustaining treatment (Koop & Grant, 1986; Lynn, 1986). Thus, a policy of leaving life-sustaining treatment plans to the discretion of the physician–patient relationship may not provide adequate oversight for vulnerable patients.

Second, there is a tension between respect for patient autonomy and respect for health care facilities' missions. A patient's unique beliefs can and often do diverge from the customary sectarian position and from an institution's view of its health care mission. Differences between a patient's preferences and a facility's mission are not a simple threat to patient autonomy; rather, they reflect the engagement of the equally respected views of a patient and a community of persons who have joined together to provide health care in a manner consonant with their moral views. If moral communities are to be able to operate institutions that reflect their values and serve the interests of those patients especially inclined to seek them out, an accommodation on this issue that provides for mutually voluntary relationships between patients and health care facilities will be needed (Ezekiel, 1988b).

Public policy could preemptively solve the difficulties raised by contending public interests by dispensing with some interests or by arranging them in a rigid hierarchy. For example, society could compel health care facilities to defer to any patient's or surrogate's wish. This solution, however, would undermine health care communities that wished to pursue missions distinguishable from any patient's personal preferences. The complexities and tensions that emerge from the diverse responsibilities of health care facilities signal important competing values. Hopefully this debate and these tensions will not be preempted.

PROTOCOLS AND CLINICAL PRACTICES

The primary objective of health facility protocols is to improve the clinical practices of decision making and treatment-plan implementation (Figure 2.1). Ethical and legal consensus about principles for proper decision making and treatment-plan implementation was partly created, and certainly synthesized, by the 1983 President's Commission, and is well described in a variety of ethics texts and review articles (see Appendix V for texts; significant summaries in the periodical literature include: Perkins, 1986, Ruark & Raffin, 1988; Wanzer et al., 1984). Essential elements of this consensus are summarized in Table 2.1.

To the end of good decision making, protocols should aim to create an informed staff who are aware of and support principles to guide good clinical practices. Presumably, clinical decision making will improve if staff uncertainty and misconceptions are addressed and staff are aware of a conceptual and procedural process for good decision making. Protocol content with regard to decision making is discussed in Chapter 7.

To the end of good treatment-plan implementation, protocols should promote explicit accountability for treatment plans and provide reliable procedures for implementing treatment decisions. Requirements for documentation promote accountability and deliberative treatment-plan construction. Protocols should minimize treatment misunderstandings by providing concise definitions of terminology and procedures. Protocols should try to prevent unacceptable practices, such as intentionally ineffective resuscitative efforts ("slow codes"), and should offer instead procedures that address clinical situations that might have led to such actions (Hastings Center, 1987). Some propose that protocols also promote empathy toward dying patients by articulating positive treatment goals (such as palliation, sensory enhancement, or social relationships) when life-sustaining treatments are no longer possible or desired. Provisions for treatment-plan implementation are examined in Chapter 8.

Protocols should also serve as frameworks for quality assurance monitoring of clinical practices involving the elective use of life-sustaining treatments. To this end, procedures should be established to provide for regularly reviewing the protocol to improve to reflect new legal developments or to address identified problems in clinical practices. Quality-assurance audits are discussed in Chapter 4.

TABLE 2.1   Decision-Making Principles for Life-Sustaining Treatments

1. Health care professionals should act to promote a patient's well being by promoting an evaluation of the benefits and burdens of therapy from the patient's perspective, and by providing care in a manner that conforms to the ethics of their profession and its standards of practice.

2. Patients have a right to make important decisions about their lives and about medical treatment for themselves.

3. Health care professionals should not be compelled to violate their personal ethical or religious convictions in the course of providing health care.

4. In some circumstances, the claims of justice or equity may constrain patient care or patient's choices as a matter of social policy.

5. The primary health care professional should conduct an evaluation of the patient's current medical condition as a foundation for all treatment decisions. This evaluation should seek to determine the diagnosis, the prognosis, the benefits, and the burdens of the treatment options, the patient's preferences, and whether there are concerned persons who are available to participate in decision making process.

6. The primary health care professional (with appropriate consultation) is responsible for assessing decisional capacity and, if it is impaired, for identifying a surrogate decision maker who is most able and willing to represent the patient's interests.

7. The primary health care professional is responsible for conducting a discussion of treatment options with the patient (or proxies if the patient lacks decisional capacity) and concerned others (within the scope of the patient's request for confidentiality).

8. Treatment decisions should be made by the patient whenever possible. If the patient is not capable of making decisions, decisions should be made according to advance directives or though a considered reflection on the patient's previously stated values. If a conscientious effort is unable to determine the patient's preferences, surrogate decision makers may make treatment decisions through best-interest or reasonable-persons standards within the bounds of accepted medical practice. Treatment futility or the irreversible loss of consciousness ordinarily weigh against the use of life-sustaining treatments.

9. The primary health care professional should document the treatment plan in a way that ensures that it is accurately implemented and that patient (or proxy) and health professional accountability for treatment decisions is maintained

10. The primary health care professional is responsible for conducting an ongoing review of the continued propriety of the treatment plan and its modification according to changing medical circumstances or patient preferences.

Source: Adapted from Hastings Center, 1987.

There are few studies of protocols' effects on clinical practices. Two studies found an increase in the use and in the understanding of DNR orders after the introduction of a DNR protocol (Bedell, Pelle, Cleary, & Maher, 1986; Quill, Stankaitis & Krause, 1986). However, this trend may have reflected an established social trend rather than the direct effect of the protocol itself. One report of the introduction of a hospital DNR protocol found that hospital staff read protocols and felt that they were helpful by clarifying the processes of making and implementing decisions to withhold life-sustaining treatment and by giving permission for more open dialogue about these issues (McPhail, Moore, O'Connor, & Woodward, 1981). This confirms anecdotal experience (Davila, Boisaubin, & Sears, 1986; Levenson et al., 1981). Other studies have found that protocols can control the use of aggressive emergency care while ensuring that attentive physician care continues (Arena, Perlin, & Turnbull, 1980; Mott & Barker, 1988; Quill et al., 1986).

The effect of protocols on the patient–physician encounter is not clear. Physicians often do not involve patients in decisions to withhold resuscitation (Bedell & Delbanco, 1984; Bedell et al., 1986; Evans & Brody, 1985; Ireland & Puri, 1983; Schwartz & Reilly, 1986; Uhlmann, McDonald, & Inui, 1984b; Witte, 1984; Youngner, Lewandowski, McClish, et al., 1985; Zimmerman et al., 1986). Treatment plans based on DNR orders often withhold a variety of other therapies, even though these collateral decisions are not documented in the medical chart (LaPuma et al., 1988b; Uhlmann et al., 1984). It is not clear whether a DNR order does (Bedell et al., 1986; Lipton, 1986; Schwartz & Reilly, 1986) or does not (Charlson et al., 1986; Lipton, 1988; Quill et al., 1986; Youngner et al., 1985) result in inappropriately reduced treatment of other kinds. Volicer has reported that families and patients can come to agreements regarding categories of treatment plans for demented persons (Volicer, 1986). Additional research is needed to determine the best way to design protocols, improve staff education, and ultimately to improve treatment planning with regard to life-sustaining treatments.

There has been relatively little criticism of the emerging consensus in favor of the general adoption of protocols to improve clinical practices, especially considering the unproven benefits of these protocols. Neonatalogists report that inflexible legal standards for decision making processes adversely affect treatment decisions (Tomlinson & Brody, 1988). Others report that health care staff believe that protocols are not needed, will have no effect on health care (Van Eys et al., 1986), and abridge physicians' prerogatives (McPhail et al., 1981; Glasser, Zweibel, & Cassel, 1988). Some experts have discounted fears that protocols will increase patients' anguish (Bedell & Delbanco, 1984; Lo & Steinbrook, 1983; Spencer, 1979; Van Scoy-Mosher, 1982) and bureaucratize practice. Kass argues that such protocols are an attempt to engineer rather than inculcate values into practice (Kass, 1985). It is also possible that procedures for limiting life-sustaining treatment might ratify paternalistic professional biases (Fox & Lipton, 1983), as is the case with nursing home protocols that omit any mention of patient autonomy (Miles & Ryden, 1985). Some fear that a poorly written protocol may adversely affect the care of vulnerable patients (Hoyt & Davies, 1986; Koop & Grant, 1986). Clearly additional research on these questions is needed.

Patients' views on these protocols have not been directly surveyed. Public opinion polls have shown strong and consistent support for shared decision making and advance directives for life-sustaining treatments (President's Commission, 1982; Society for the Right to Die, 1987). Presumably this approval means that patients would support health facility protocols that attempted to promote these practices.

CONCLUSION

The final objective of health care facility protocols is to improve patient care. This complex task needs to be grounded in a thorough understanding of what institutional and professional duties and procedures are summoned in these practices. From this understanding, protocols can promote decision making and treatment practices that educate staff, coordinate complex procedures, and establish a framework for identifying and addressing clinical problems.

PART II
Protocol Development and Implementation

CHAPTER 3
Protocol Development

The process of creating a protocol to address the elective use of life-sustaining treatments has three phases: recognizing the need for a protocol, creating and educating a group to draft the protocol, and the drafting of the protocol.

RECOGNIZING THE NEED FOR PROTOCOLS

The impetus for creating a protocol to address life-sustaining treatments can arise from diverse personal interests within the facility, as well as from institutional concerns (Halligan & Hamel, 1985; Levenson, List, & Zaw-Win, 1981; McPhail, Moore, O'Connor, & Woodward, 1981; Van Eys, Bowen, & Alt, 1986). Many protocols arise from the efforts of informed staff or administrators, sometimes responding to controversial public cases, who want to improve care in their facilities. Some arise when staff are troubled by a situation within the facility that may involve intrafamily conflicts or the care of a patient who is especially well known to the facility. Some protocols arise from interstaff tensions, such as when nurses press for protocols after a physician has verbally given a DNR order, but will not write it in the medical record.

Protocols are also initiated in response to larger institutional pressures. Models proposed by the central administrations of large health care systems, such as the Veterans Administration, have stimulated the development of local protocols (Veterans Administration, 1984). Recently issued

Joint Commission accrediting standards for hospitals and nursing homes (Appendix III) will undoubtedly lead additional facilities to develop protocols (Burmeister, 1986; Joint Commission, 1987; Chapter 2). Protocols have also been created as a form of risk management to help ensure that clinical practice conforms to public policies (Brenner & Gerken, 1986; Kapp, 1987). Other protocols have been developed in response to direct legal requirements. New York state now requires hospitals and nursing homes to develop and implement DNR protocols (New York State Task Force, 1987). Other states have patients' rights and advance directive legislation that mandates or encourages health care facilities to develop protocols (Concern for Dying, 1987; HCFA, 1979). Some states, such as Illinois, permit nursing homes to withhold resuscitation only when the facility has a protocol that stipulates the procedures to be followed in reaching and recording such a decision (Illinois DPH, 1979). Some protocols originate as nursing homes try to coordinate their DNR procedures with those of ambulance services.

The genesis of protocols in a single staff group (i.e., lawyers, nurses, administrators, or physicians) can adversely affect protocol development. Parochial staff views can be emphasized in a way that is counterproductive, especially if the concern originates in a perception that other groups are improperly addressing the elective use of life-sustaining treatments (Halligan & Hamel, 1985). Thus, clinicians might author protocols without fully understanding the legal obligations of the facility vis-à-vis vulnerable adults. The mistaken view, for example, that living wills are illegal unless specifically enacted by the state legislature, can be an important barrier to the use of advance directives (Byrne, 1982; Kapp, 1987). Likewise, protocols written at the behest of administrators may reflect a risk-management agenda that is insensitive to the complexities of common and urgent clinical dilemmas. Regardless of where or why protocol drafting is started, the facility should try to create a multidisciplinary drafting process.

THE PROTOCOL DRAFTING GROUP

Protocol drafting groups should allow multidisciplinary collaboration among nurses, social workers, physicians, administrators, and lawyers (American Hospital Association, 1985; Lo, 1987). A diverse drafting group can draw on the varied expertise of these professional groups, all of which will be affected by the protocol. A multidisciplinary group also provides an excellent forum where different perspectives can be thoughtfully addressed in inclusive protocols. Nurses and physicians, for instance, may have differing emotional and moral conclusions about the use of life-sustaining treatments (Frampton & Mayewski, 1987; Gramelspacher, Howell, & Young, 1986; Levenson et al.,

1981; Wolff et al., 1985). A multidisciplinary drafting group will be most able to create procedures that can be practically incorporated into the daily routines of various professionals. Finally, the process of multidisciplinary drafting creates a group of staff who are uniquely qualified and capable of introducing and interpreting the protocol to their colleagues and thereby facilitating its implementation.

Creating and sustaining multidisciplinary forums to author health care facility protocols for decisions about life-sustaining treatments can be difficult. Many clinicians do not enjoy committee work. Crowded schedules work against sustained committee assignments. The less frequent presence of attending physicians in nursing homes can make collaboration especially difficult in that setting. Interprofessional tensions and different styles of communication can further hinder communication among lawyers, administrators, and clinicians (Lo, 1987). Lack of administrative support for staff education, for staff time, or for the drafting process itself can demoralize drafting groups (American Hospital Association, 1985).

Committed leadership from within the health care facility can motivate staff to participate in protocol drafting despite these barriers. The problems these protocols address are common, vexing, and important to nearly all clinicians. Clinical ethics is an intrinsically interesting topic that engages the core of people's beliefs and primary motivations for entering the profession. Rather than stressing the difficult and often intractable legal and administrative aspects of medical ethical problems, health facility leadership should frame the task of protocol drafting and implementation as a central task of professional patient care responsibilities. By stressing the professional and collegial nature of this task, health facility leadership can encourage staff members to become committed to the process of protocol drafting.

At a minimum, protocol-drafting groups should include a physician, nurse, social worker, cleric, lawyer, and administrator (Cranford & Ashley, 1986; Doudera & Peters, 1982; Glasser, Zweibel, & Cassel, 1988; Lynn, 1982; Miles & Ryden, 1985). Other staff members may be added because of their personal interests or skills, or to promote intrafacility communication. The facility's lawyer should be involved in the entire process of protocol drafting so that he or she becomes familiar with clinical needs, can review the emerging case and statutory law in this field with clinicians (Kapp, 1985), and can help address staff misperceptions about legal liability (Brenner & Gerken, 1988). Likewise, health care facility administrators who are removed from daily bedside concerns should participate in the drafting process to better understand how the facility's interests apply to daily clinical realities. New accrediting standards require that the chief administrator be involved in drafting a protocol (Joint Commission, 1987). This can include explaining

the protocol to the governing board, securing their approval, and implementing the protocol.

The relative contributions of staff groups to protocol drafting will vary
with the facility and with the interests of staff members. In hospitals, physicians often play a dominant role, though nurses, social workers, and clergy
have chaired such committees as well. In nursing homes, nurses are more
familiar with the day to day clinical life of patients and have greater influence
on treatment plans, even though the physician remains ultimately responsible for medical orders. Nurses and social workers play a greater leadership
role in drafting nursing home protocols (Glasser, Zweibel, & Cassel, 1988;
Miles & Ryden, 1985). Leadership for a drafting group may also come from
an administrator or a "bioethically" sensitive lawyer (Kapp, 1985).

Health care facilities have created several kinds of protocol drafting
groups. Ethics committees often assume this task (Bayley & Doudera, 1986;
Cranford & Doudera, 1984; ,Lo, 1987; Lynn, 1984; President's Commission,
1983), and conversely, protocol drafting committees have evolved into ethics
committee in many facilities.* Multidisciplinary patient-care conferences are
another forum from which protocols can emerge if time is reserved from the
day-to-day minutiae of patient care to engage in this task. Ad hoc protocol
drafting committees or task forces have also been convened (Halligan &
Hamel, 1985, Van Eys et al., 1981). Utilization-review committees, whose
primary agenda is cost containment, should not be recruited for this purpose, in that cost containment and patient advocacy pose a potential conflict
of interest.

Protocol-drafting groups often begin their task without being specifically
empowered to do so by the governing board of the facility. For such groups,
administrative standing or ratification of the protocol by the chief of staff,
director of nursing, or board of trustees may come later, when the group's
purpose and track record is clearer. In some facilities, the task of protocol
drafting is formally assigned to a committee that reports to the director of
the facility, the director of the medical staff, or director of nursing. New Joint
Commission standards require that nursing home and hospital protocols for
decisions about resuscitation be ratified by the highest governing board of
the facility (Joint Commission, 1987; see Appendix III). The practice in some

---

* Institutional ethics committees are multidisciplinary bodies whose purpose is to assist hospital and nursing home practitioners in resolving complex ethical decisions by providing staff
education, and assisting with policy development and case consultation (Allen & Miles, 1987;
Brown, Henteloff, Baraka, & Rowe, 1987; Cassel et al., 1986). Government panels (President's
Commission, 1983) and professional associations (Committee on Ethics and Medical-Legal
Affairs, 1985; Judicial Council, 1985; American Hospital Association, 1984) have encouraged
the formation of ethics committees. The purposes, uses, and forms of ethics committees have
been discussed in several excellent reviews (Cranford & Doudera, 1984; President's Commission, 1983; Rosner, 1985).

facilities of having only protocols endorsed by a medical staff or department of nursing is no longer sufficient by Joint Commission standards; the need for an interdepartmental protocol is another potent reason for multidisciplinary drafting groups.

THE PROTOCOL DRAFTING PROCESS

Although there has been little research as to how individual health care facilities actually draft these protocols (Lo, 1987), anecdotal experiences identify several features of the drafting process (Halligan & Hamel, 1985; Levenson et al., 1981, McPhail et al., 1981; Van Eys et al., 1986). Ethics committees usually attempt protocol drafting before they perform case consultations (Brown, Miles, & Aroskar, 1987; Glasser, Zweibel, & Cassel, 1988). The group often begins by exploring the reasons (and emotions) that led to the institutional (and personal) interest in a protocol. After several meetings, members may become discouraged at the apparent intractability of the problems, as ambitious expectations for protocol development and resolution of perceived problems give way to a deeper understanding of the problems. At this critical juncture, leadership should focus committee members' efforts on acquiring education that will serve as a foundation for protocol drafting or ethics consultations.

The agenda for, or duration of, committee education will vary greatly depending on the committee's task and its members' backgrounds. Protocol authors should familiarize themselves with a standard text in medical ethics. (See Appendix V for a suggested list.) Clinical and legal staff should jointly review case law and statutory law in treatment decision making, informed consent, termination of treatment, advance directives, the care of vulnerable or incompetent adults, patient rights, and brain death, as well as other topics related to their facility's needs. Building on this base of legal and ethical knowledge, clinical ethics case discussions can be an excellent way to explore the complex nature of the clinical problems (Veatch, 1977; see Appendix V for selected bioethics literature). Such cases might be drawn from the literature rather than from the facility, so that the discussion does not unduly focus on local personalities. If protocols are to address the use of emergency medical services or state guardians, these bodies' procedures should be reviewed with those responsible for these services. Some facilities will employ consultants, such as outside ethicists, lawyers with expertise on these questions, diocesan authorities, or disability advocates, to assist in protocol drafting (Hoyt & Davies, 1986). The facility should expect to support the allocation of staff time to this process and to bear the costs of educational materials, staff education, and consultants.

Protocol drafters often examine models or protocols from other facilities in order to guide their own protocol drafting process. Models are advisory documents that are developed by institutions claiming special expertise or authority in order to assist health care facilities in developing their own protocols or guidelines. A variety of models are available including those of American Hospital Association, 1985; Bar Association, 1983; Hastings Center, 1987; Hoyt & Davies, 1984, 1986; Joint Commission, 1987; Medical Society, 1983; Minnesota Medical, 1983; Task Force, 1984; Veterans Administration, 1984; Uhlmann et al., 1987; Wanzer et al., 1984, as well as the individual facility protocols cited throughout this book.*

Models are often amended before being adopted at a given facility. They may be modified to take into account the special capabilities, administrative structure, procedures, or mission of a facility. Models are also modified to conform to local guardianship procedures, emergency medical systems procedures, and local usages of key terms (e.g., DNR). Existing models or examples for DNR protocols may need to be amended to conform to new Joint Commission standards or other regulatory or accrediting networks to which the facility is accountable.

Adaptation of models is more than simply fitting the model to a facility. Amending a model is a part of the process of staff education and helps the diverse membership of the drafting group come to understand the implications of the model for their own facility's needs, procedures, and concerns. Adapting a model is a way by which health care staff come to "own" the provisions of the protocol and become committed to its implementation (Van Eys et al., 1986). Thus, models should be debated, not merely explained. Amendments—even to a well regarded model—should be encouraged, challenged, and passed if they can be successfully defended by an informed drafting committee.

---

* Models are an effective way for knowledgeable and prestigious bodies to disseminate expertise. A model DNR policy developed by a state medical association (Minnesota Medical Association, 1983; Miles et al., 1982) was copied by several other state medical associations (Bar Association, 1983; Medical Society of the State of New York, 1983; Medical Association, 1983) and incorporated into many hospital policies (Miles & Moldow, 1984, 1985).

Authors of models should anticipate that the model will be adapted by individual facilities. The greater the diversity of the facilities to which the model is addressed, the greater the modification of the model. A nursing-home chain operating within a single state should be able to write a model that can be readily adopted by its facilities, if there is sufficient involvement of clinicians in the drafting so that the model is cognizant of clinical realities. Such models might provide for local flexibility in the designation of staff to coordinate staff education or ethics committees according to local talents and interests. Models that address a diverse universe of facilities should anticipate the need for substantial local amendment. Such models might well include menus of optional provisions to encourage adaptation of an individual policy (Minnesota Hospital Association, 1986).

Most protocols go through many drafts that are circulated to staff out-side of the drafting committee. Drafts should be circulated to clinical super-visors and other key personnel as well as to a diverse group of clinical staff for comments and revisions before the final protocol is adopted (McPhail et al., 1981). Out of this process of intrafacility discussion, some facilities have adopted initial statements of principle that reflect a foundational consensus as to how to address decisions to limit treatment (Halligan & Hamel, 1985; Van Eys et al., 1986). Presumably, more prescriptive procedural protocols can be based on these principles. It is hoped that intra-facility discussion of protocol drafts will lead to a protocol that is understood, workable, and respected. It also may be crucial to supporting a later institutional claim that the principles and procedures in the protocol represents the moral position of staff or the facility, as is discussed in Chapter 2.

CONCLUSION

Drafting a protocol is a collaborative process that entails the integration of a diverse set of personal, professional, and institutional concerns. The recog-nition of the need for an improved institutional response to the elective use of life-sustaining treatments may arise in one staff or administrative con-stituency. The drafting process may profit from consultation with experts and models from outside the facility. Ultimately, however, protocols work to the degree that staff understand their rationale, are convinced of their value, and are able to incorporate their provisions into complex, multidisci-plinary, institutional health care practices.

CHAPTER 4
Protocol Implementation

Protocols to address the elective use of life-sustaining treatments are one element of an institution's effort to address perennially difficult issues of the elective use of life-sustaining treatments. By themselves, administrative protocols can not resolve these problems and will have little impact on clinical practices. Protocols should go hand-in-hand with ongoing administrative support to improve clinical practices, staff education, and ongoing review of the quality of care.

ADMINISTRATIVE SUPPORT

Little is written about health care facility administrators' duties vis-à-vis the implementation of a response to the elective use of life-sustaining treatments (American Hospital Association, 1984; Joint Commission, 1987; Kapp, 1987). Administrators should support forums for collaboration among nurses, social workers, physicians, administrators, and lawyers to create and implement these protocols. Funds, time, and administrative support are needed to train staff as ethics consultants or to serve on ethics committees to assist other staff with difficult individual cases (Cranford & Doudera, 1984; Hosford, 1986). Ongoing inservice training in ethics and procedural duties should be provided. The facility might make one or more of the bioethics journals available (see Appendix V for a selected listing) or send staff to professional-education conferences that address these issues.

Administrative support will also be required to implement new procedures. Advance directives should be made available to clinical staff for distribution to patients. Medical records may have to be structured to convey information about treatment objectives and preferences (see Part III). Interagency agreements will be needed to provide for effective coordination of treatment plans with EMS services during interfacility transfers (Hastings Center, 1987; Miles & Crimmins, 1985). Practical mechanisms should be established to comply with mandated reporting or consulting relationships with guardian's offices.

STAFF EDUCATION

The multidisciplinary protocol-drafting process sets the stage for protocol implementation and is a foundation for staff education. Hopefully, the drafting group will have created a core group of clinical and administrative staff who understand the clinical, ethical, and legal rationale for the protocol. Circulated drafts have introduced the principles upon which the protocol is based and the proposed procedures to address them. Clinicians, administrators, and lawyers have become familiar with the clinical and ethical context of decisions about life-sustaining treatments and with procedures (e.g., living wills, special medical records, or ethics committees) that can be used to improve clinical practices.

Staff should be familiarized with the protocol (Halligan & Hamel, 1985; McPhail et al., 1981; Van Eys et al., 1986). Protocol drafters should present the document to staff, and copies of the protocol should be distributed. Meetings should be scheduled so that night or on-call staff, who will implement many orders during medical emergencies, can also attend and do not have to rely on tape recordings or minutes of staff meetings. Case studies illustrating the process, from decision making to the construction of treatment plans and medical orders, to treatment implementation, can promote understanding of the use of the protocols. Sample medical records with completed documentation can also be helpful. One hospital has developed a staff pamphlet that informs staff how to address ethics conflicts in their practice (St. Joseph's, 1984e). Questions and reservations about the protocol should be elicited and carefully considered. One innovative hospital has successfully implemented a supportive-care team to assist health care staff in caring for dying or hopelessly ill persons (Carlson, Devich, & Frank, 1988).

Although many staff will welcome efforts to address the use of life-sustaining treatment, some may challenge the drafter's legal, medical, or administrative expertise. They might view the requirement for signed records of decisions to withhold treatment as increasing legal liability and paper work (Grand Jury, 1985; McPhail et al., 1981). They might suggest that the protocol unduly emphasizes the concerns of a particular staff group (Halligan & Hamel, 1985), or assert that the protocol is irrelevant to clinical needs (Van Eys et al., 1986). These challenges will be more easily addressed if drafters of diverse competencies are able to describe a credible process of self-education and establish the authority from which they have derived the protocol (Ruark & Raffin, 1988). The clinicians, administrators, and lawyers in the drafting group should be able to defend the protocol from the perspective of their work and from what they have learned from other disciplines during the drafting process.

Some staff may maintain that a protocol will constrain professional discretion or bind staff to morally objectionable views of health care. There are several responses to these objections. First, the concept of shared treatment decisions between responsible professionals and informed, consenting patients is a widely accepted medical, social, legal, and philosophical ideal—not a radical innovation. Second, within this decision-making theory, protocols do not dictate the outcome of the clinical decision-making relationship, but in the main, rather, propose a process for the treatment planning. Procedural requirements for deliberative decision making, accurate implementation, and firm accountability for treatment plans are all ways intended to decrease misunderstandings and mistakes, and thus might be viewed as decreasing legal risks. Finally, by allowing clinicians to excuse themselves from objectionable treatment preferences (see Part III), protocols preserve the professional's conscience as they promote patient autonomy. Some observers of debates over the moral foundations of protocols have noted that even contradictory views of moral health care may not preclude agreement on the course of action to take in a given situation (Toulmin, 1981). Thus, case discussions, rather than extended discussions of ethical principles, should help focus staff education, assure its clinical relevance, and lead to the broadest possible consensus. A number of texts with sample cases are available (see Appendix V).

There should be continuing staff education on the elective use of life-sustaining treatments. New clinical problems and an evolving understanding of the complexities of the elective use of life-sustaining treatment will require continuing discussion and improvement of these protocols. Procedures should also be established to educate newly hired staff.

QUALITY ASSURANCE

Facilities should establish quality-assurance mechanisms to monitor and modify the elective use of life-sustaining treatments. Little is known about the use of quality-assurance procedures to examine the elective use of life-sustaining treatment (Halligan & Hamel, 1985; Hoyt & Davies, 1986; Integrate QA, 1987). "Quality care" encompasses the quality of decision making, the overutilization and underutilization of life-sustaining treatments, and the consequences of clinical practices. The difficulty defining, let alone achieving, ideal clinical practices for the elective use of life-sustaining treatments does not exempt administrators from a duty to address readily identifiable deficiencies in clinical practice (Brook, 1977). The objectives of promoting patient autonomy, protecting vulnerable persons, accommodating staff's moral convictions, conforming to laws, and ensuring accountable and accurate treatment-plan implementation could well serve as the foundation for a quality-assurance program (Chapter 2).

Donabedian's widely accepted tripartite framework of *structure*, *process*, and *outcome* for quality assessment suggests an approach to monitoring the implementation of these protocols (Donabedian, 1969). This model assumes that better *structures* and *processes* will result in better patient care *outcomes*.

Structural assessment evaluates the settings and instruments for the provision of care. In this context, structures include administrative supports to improve clinical practices. Structural audits might periodically evaluate whether the protocol conforms to law, regulations, and Joint Commission accrediting standards (1987). A facility might wish to set its own more stringent standards for structural assessment, including whether it addresses the most common clinical situations and the known problem areas of clinical practices (Rutstein, 1976). Audits might also address the structure of ethics committees, their mission statement, composition, meetings, minutes, and educational services. Audits might evaluate the ongoing staff education programs, including the way that staff are informed of the protocol and receive a certain minimum of inservice training in the elective use of life-sustaining treatments. Audits might also evaluate the availability of advance directives, interfacility transfer forms, and so forth.

Process assessments evaluate the clinical practices, which in this context include decision making and treatment-plan implementation. Process audits might monitor whether or not the record shows that patients and their families were informed of and participated in treatment planning. Process audits might also evaluate treatment practices, such as whether patients who died without resuscitation in fact had orders to withhold resuscitation.

Outcome assessments evaluate health outcomes and patient satisfaction with care. Further research is needed to determine reasonable quality-assurance measures to assess the outcomes of withholding or withdrawing life-sustaining interventions. Patient or family satisfaction with the planning process might be one outcome that could be assessed.

Simple quality-assurance methods might include committee review of "problem" cases or chart sampling (especially of patients with orders to limit treatment or of patients who have died). Such auditing could evaluate: documentation of treatment plans that involve decisions to withhold or provide life-sustaining treatments, the accuracy of DNR implementation, whether patients or proxies are involved in treatment planning, the distribution and use of living wills, and the like. The results of audits should be relayed to those responsible for protocol amendments or staff education in order to improve the delivery of care in light of the institution's responsibilities.

CONCLUSION

Implementing protocols for the elective use of life-sustaining treatments is a complex and ongoing administrative responsibility. This task includes providing administrative support for new types of medical charting and advance directives. It entails ensuring that staff have access to ethical and legal expertise. An ongoing process of staff education should convey needed information and foster an interdisciplinary dialogue so that multidisciplinary decision making and treatment-plan implementation can occur. Fully implementing these protocols includes assessing the adequacy of the administrative support for these problematic clinical practices and assessing the quality of the care that is finally rendered.

PART III
Protocol Content

CHAPTER 5
Protocol Formats

Protocol drafters face a bewildering task. Variations on protocol design are infinite. The effects of protocol design on clinical practices are not clear. Each facility's patients, treatment issues, and administrative framework seem to require a unique protocol design. Protocol drafters must somehow collate a diverse body of knowledge about medical ethics, clinical practices, and practical administrative procedures. The complexities of this task should be approached with a clear focus on patients' clinical needs.

CASE SAMPLES AND PROTOCOL DESIGN

Protocols should be designed to address common and troubling clinical situations. Although no protocol can anticipate every possible situation, a protocol should be flexible enough to respond to any patient's needs, if only by establishing a special procedure for expert consideration of difficult and novel questions. Case studies, resembling common clinical situations in the facility, can provide a useful point of reference for a developing protocol. The following cases are used in discussions of protocol provisions in the subsequent chapters of this book. We also will refer to these cases as we consider designs for institutional frameworks that promote good treatment planning and implementation. (See Table 5.1.)

William Anderson, 82 years old, lives in the intermediate care section of Willow Rest Nursing Home. He has moderately severe emphysema, has had

TABLE 5.1   The Goals and Scope of Policies

To promote good decision making by:
  Enhancing patient autonomy
  Protecting vulnerable patients
  Promoting institutional missions
  Excusing staff with conscientious objections
  Separating financial interests from treatment decision making
  Providing assistance with complex decisions

To promote good treatment plan implementation by:
  Establishing presumptions in favor of treatment
  Maintaining accountability of staff for decisions and their implementation
  Providing for reliable communication of the treatment plan
  Coordinating care with other institutions involved in patient care

two myocardial infarctions, and one leg amputated because of arterial in-sufficiency. He has no family, but is active in the social life of the facility. He wishes to categorically decline resuscitation in the event of a cardiac arrest. He wants all life-sustaining therapies withheld if "I am a vegetable," and no longer able to socially interact with other persons. Aside from these prefer-ences, he wants to continue to receive aggressive life-prolonging care or emergency treatment of suffering from potentially lethal conditions, such as pulmonary edema. He is also interested in having his body used for medical research or transplantation.

Rita Jackson is 64 years old; she is aphasic and hemiplegic from a stroke 2 years earlier. Because she is incontinent of urine and dependent in all activities of her daily life, she resides in the skilled section of Willow Rest, a private nursing home, at public expense. She is unable to communicate by speech, writing, or gesture. After intensive physical therapy, she is dependent on others for assistance in transferring to a wheelchair. She enjoys food, grooming, and the companionship of the nursing aides. No family come to visit.

Susan Swift is a 47 year-old woman with widely metastatic cancer that has progressed despite surgery, chemotherapy, and radiation. She has just been admitted to Mill Town Community Hospital by her family who have been caring for her at home. She had been under the care of an oncologist who provided technically expert care but with whom she had never felt comfortable discussing what would happen after treatment could no longer stay the tumor. On this admission, the oncologist has told the family to return her to the care of her family physician who has not seen her for 2 years.

  The hospital nurses know the patient from many earlier admissions for radiation and chemotherapy. For the last year, Ms. Swift has told her family and nurses that the only reason that she has taken chemotherapy is to relieve the pain of the deposits of cancer in her bones. She did not believe that it would prevent her from dying of this cancer. She is now obtunded and appears to be in some pain. The tumors have spread throughout her lungs, liver, and skeleton. No remediable electrolyte abnormality or brain lesion is causing her depressed level of consciousness. Her husband, who has been with her on her previous admissions, accompanies her.

Walter Jones is an outpatient with AIDS. He is aware of the course of his disease and fears that he will lose his ability to reason. Despite his physician's reservations, he wants all life-prolonging measures taken, including endotracheal intubation, CPR, and antibiotics. But he is strongly opposed to life-prolonging care if he should irreversibly lose his ability to reason. He is estranged from his family who live in the same town as he does. Mr. Jones wishes to be sure his own preferences are honored and asks that his closest friend and long time lover be allowed to speak on his behalf in the future. His friend understands and supports Mr. Jones' views and is willing to act as a surrogate.

Dr. Ruth Steinberg is medical director of Shalom Home, a nursing home created and supported by an Orthodox synagogue. Shalom Home mainly admits elderly members of the congregation, but has also admitted a few noncongregants as well. Dr. Steinberg encourages her staff to reflect on the ethical aspects of their work in light of the Jewish traditions. Dr. Steinberg, together with her staff and the rabbi for the synagogue and Shalom Home, are aware of recent developments with regard to the discontinuation of nourishment. They have concluded that, in light of the views of their faith, a final decision about whether or not to permit discontinuation of nourishment of a patient within the facility should be made by an ethics committee chaired by the rabbi. Although this is not an immediate clinical issue in their facility, they do not want eventually to be compelled, against their moral laws, to participate in the withholding of nourishment from a resident.

PROTOCOL VOICE

Administrative protocols can speak in several voices. They may inform, suggest, recommend, persuade, exhort, or command. They may define what is forbidden, what is minimally acceptable, what is desirable, or what is ideal. We propose that protocol provisions may be considered as having three major kinds of voice (see Table 5.2). The *policy voice* mandates certain standards of acceptable conduct. The *guideline voice* recommends principles for conduct to which practitioners should strive but may not fully attain. The *working-paper* voice is mainly used in draft documents that are used to locate

TABLE 5.2   Protocol Voices

	Minimal standards	Ideal standards
Mandating	Policy voice	Prophetic voice
Suggesting	Working paper	Guideline voice

a consensus. The *prophetic voice*, which commands the ideal, is not considered here (Gustafson, 1988).

The hallmark of the policy voice is its prescriptive language. The policy voice establishes essential or minimally acceptable standards of conduct. Thus, "the physician must write the DNR order in the permanent medical record," is a policy statement. The policy voice is used to state fundamental institutional precepts, to assign responsibility, and to detail procedures for treatment implementation.

The guideline voice is an advisory rather than a prescriptive voice. The provisional nature of the guideline voice suits it to suggesting approaches to complex decisions or proposing ideals to help organize difficult clinical situations. Guidelines can be used to elaborate on how principles such as patient autonomy can be applied to clinical practice or to recommend a counseling approach for discussing the elective use of life-sustaining treatment. Thus, "decisions for cognitively impaired patients should, as closely as possible, reflect the patient's own point of view" states a goal to which advance planning aspires while implicitly recognizing that this may be an incompletely attainable ideal in clinical practice. The guideline voice is a gentle voice that inculcates values, rather than legislate solutions (Kass, 1985; Siegler, 1981; President's Commission, 1982).

Draft protocols might be written in a working-paper voice. Working papers might discuss approaches to complex clinical problems and consider alternatives for procedures or principles. Working papers can be most useful when consensus on standards of practice is still emerging. Thus, working papers might address problems of competing moral claims (e.g., how is procedural protection for vulnerable patients to be reconciled with not obstructing patient autonomy?). Working papers should be inclusive, including clear statements of contending positions and highlighting areas of disagreement and common ground. The working-paper voice is an invitation to further reflection and research (Halligan & Hamel, 1985).

The different voices of policies, guidelines, and working papers are tools for creating a consensus upon which a protocol can rest. In creating this consensus, the exploratory nature of a working paper is a strength, a premature assertion can preempt a constructive debate of these complex issues.

Eventually, the working voice must give way to commitments: minimal standards and ideals for clinical practices. There will be issues, such as the discontinuation of invasive nourishment, where consensus will not be possible. These areas should not stop the development of a protocol on areas where consensus exists. Successful protocols should be designed with an eye to what is possible and incrementally better, rather than what is ultimately envisaged or seems intellectually complete.

Policy and guideline voices are often combined in single protocols (Beth Israel, 1983; Meisel et al., 1986; Miles, Cranford, & Schultz, 1982). In such documents, the difference between these voices should be kept in mind in order to avoid using policy language where guidelines or working-paper language is more appropriate. Some policies, for example, restrict DNR orders to terminally ill persons. This misleadingly suggests that DNR orders cannot be written for non-terminally ill persons, such as Mr. Anderson or Ms. Jackson (McPhail et al., 1981; Veterans Administration, 1984).

Protocols should be written so that physicians, nurses, and social workers can understand and implement them. They should use clear, jargon-free, nonlegalistic language. A format with concise topic headings will help practitioners to locate desired information. Policies should probably be no longer than 10 to 15 pages, so that health care staff can grasp the totality of their intent and implementation. Models that are designed to address the diverse needs of many health care facilities might be somewhat longer, with the expectation that they will be shortened. Because models (such as the Veterans Administration model in Appendix IV) will usually be adapted by a facility's ethics experts, they may be somewhat more complex than finished protocols. Model designers should recognize that few staff will have had formal training in medical ethics or law. One successfully disseminated model fit on a single page (Minnesota Medical Association, 1983).

PARADIGMS FOR TREATMENT PLANS

One of the most difficult tasks for protocols is to propose a conceptual paradigm for treatment plans that selectively employ life-sustaining treatments. The treatment-plan paradigm is a tool for communicating the treatment plan between health care providers and with patients. Three paradigms are currently used: *do-not-resuscitate orders, care categories,* and *limited-treatment plans.* Each was created to answer a clinical need. Each has advantages and limitations. Each was created for a particular setting, and its usefulness and disadvantages change as it is translated to other settings.

Do-Not-Resuscitate Protocols

Do-not-resuscitate protocols are the most widely used form of protocol for elective use of a life-sustaining treatment in hospitals (Miles & Moldow, 1984; Mozdzierz & Schlesinger, 1986; Hospital Council, 1984). DNR orders permit an individual exception to a standing order to provide CPR to any patient suffering a cardiac arrest. DNR orders are commonly written on general medical wards and in intensive care units (Evans & Brody, 1985; LaPuma, Silverstein, Stocking, Boland, Siegler, 1988; Lipton, 1986; Uhlmann, MacDonald, Inui, 1984; Witte, 1984; Youngner et al., 1985). DNR orders are created by the primary physician and usually implemented by on-call staff who, because of the nature of cardiac arrest and the urgency of CPR, are unable to confer with the patient or primary physician about the desirability of CPR (Youngner, 1987). New Joint Commission standards for hospitals and nursing homes require DNR protocols in accredited facilities (see Appendix III). Many examples of DNR protocols are published (Beth Israel, 1982; City of Boston, 1983; Los Angeles, 1983; McPhail et al., 1981; Miles et al., 1982; Northwestern, 1982; Somerville Hospital, 1983; St. Joseph's, 1984a; St. Joseph's, 1984b; University of Wisconsin, 1983).

The use of standing orders to ensure that CPR is promptly and effectively given necessitates protocols for DNR orders. In the absence of a protocol, withholding CPR violates the standing order for CPR. By authorizing the DNR order, the institution legitimizes the DNR decision and creates a procedure (the signed DNR order) to simultaneously implement this decision and hold physicians accountable for it. DNR protocols also discourage, but do not eliminate (Quill, Stankaitis, & Krause, 1986) unwritten, verbally passed DNR orders. The indictment of a New York hospital where no physician would accept responsibility for an unwritten DNR order presents a compelling argument in favor of DNR protocols (Deputy Attorney, 1983; Grand Jury, 1985).

The written DNR order is a unique auditable notation of a decision to withhold a life-sustaining medical treatment. It has led to considerable research about this decision to limit a life-sustaining treatment (Bedell & Delbanco, 1984; Evans & Brody, 1985; LaPuma, 1988; Lipton, 1986; Quill et al., 1986; Office of Technology Assessment, 1987; Uhlmann, Cassel, & McDonald, 1984; Uhlmann, McDonald, Inui, 1984; Witte, 1984; Youngner et al., 1985; see also Chapter 2). The written DNR order is also an accessible chart notation for quality-assurance audits, as discussed in Chapter 4.

Since their introduction during the late 1970s, the inadequacies of DNR protocols have become increasingly evident as an emerging public consensus has accepted the idea that all life-sustaining treatments are elective. In many settings, the DNR order has become synonymous with a broader concept of limited-treatment plans, wrongly being equated with the rejection of other life-sustaining treatments (Donnelly, 1987; Ross & Pugh, 1988; Tomlinson & Brody, 1988). Clinical studies have found DNR orders being interpreted as restricting a cluster of life-sustaining treatments beyond CPR (Bedell, et al., 1986; Evans & Brody, 1985; LaPuma, Silverstein, Stocking, Boland, & Siegler, 1988; Meisel et al., 1986; Uhlmann, Cassel, McDonald, 1984). Some commentators have even proposed that DNR orders be understood as meaning that prolongation of life is no longer a treatment goal (Paris, 1982; Stevens, 1986). This misconception contributes to an inability to appreciate the variety of patient preferences and medical circumstances of patients with DNR orders (Tomlinson & Brody, 1988).

DNR protocols address a decision of limited scope, a single element in a treatment plan. Although DNR protocols provide a means to implement a decision to withhold CPR, they do not provide a means to communicate important differences between William Anderson's, Susan Swift's, or Walter Jones' treatment plans. CPR is virtually the only treatment Mr. Anderson wishes to forego, but in Mrs. Swift's case, CPR is to be withheld along with all other life-prolonging therapies. To the extent that protocols allow staff to think of Mr. Anderson and Mrs. Swift as "no-code" patients and thus allow them to receive equivalent care, protocols do a disservice that potentially endangers Mr. Anderson (Miles & Ryden, 1985). Mr. Jones' preference for CPR until it is established that he is irreversibly incapable of reasoning should be incorporated into an advance directive that would become a DNR order at some future time.

Protocols have attempted to address the confused understanding of the DNR order in several ways. Some narrowly define the DNR order as countermanding the CPR standing order (Youngner, 1987). A common definition reads, "In the event of cardiac or pulmonary arrest, no cardiopulmonary resuscitative measure will be initiated" (Minnesota Medical Association, 1983). Others emphasize that DNR should not, of itself, restrict other life-sustaining treatment or lessen the care to prevent cardiac arrest (American Hospital Association, 1985b; Hastings, 1987; Miles et al., 1982; National Conference, 1986; Office of Technology Assessment, 1987; President's Commission, 1983; Read, 1983; Veteran's Administration, 1984).

Despite the conceptual inadequacy of using DNR orders to frame limited treatment plans, DNR protocols have focused the discussion of how to design health care facility protocols. Today, DNR protocols are widely used, and are endorsed by the Joint Commission as a standard for administrative practice (see Appendix III). Nevertheless, DNR protocols are a prototype. Successors to DNR protocols will address a broad variety of life-sustaining treatments, including whether or not to use CPR as a single element in a comprehensive treatment plan (Greenlaw, 1986; Hastings Center, 1987).

Care-Category Protocols

The limited scope of DNR protocols has led to interest in protocols that address an array of life-sustaining treatments. Care-category protocols attempt to address many kinds of therapies and to simplify the complexity of endless potential treatment choices. Two types of care-category protocols have been proposed: *Treatment-category protocols* and *Goal-category protocols*.

Treatment-category protocols assign patients to one of several hierarchically stratified groups of medical treatments (Arena et al., 1980; Callahan, 1987; Committee on Policy, 1983; Clinical Care, 1976; Davila et al., 1986 Executive Committee, 1976; Levenson et al., 1981; Meisel et al., 1986; Mott et al., 1988; Quill et al., 1986; Volicer et al., 1986; Yarrows, 1987). A patient assigned to a particular category is generally ineligible for treatments that belong in the higher categories. Hospital protocols have defined categories around decisions such as DNR or admission to an intensive care unit (ICU). One typical protocol creates three categories: All But Cardiac Resuscitation, Limited Therapy (in which no new therapy is initiated), and Comfort Measures Only, in which all treatments not related to comfort and hygiene are discontinued (Meisel et al., 1986). A nursing home policy has used the decision to forego hospitalization to divide treatment levels (Levenson et al., 1981). Again, a lowest level contains only palliative therapies (see Table 5.3).

Goal-category protocols categorize management objectives rather than treatment modalities themselves (Braithwaite & Thomasma, 1986; Halligan & Hamel, 1985; Task Force, 1984). Goal categories might be defined as "palliative care only" or "prolonging life." Goal categories attempt to address the problem that a given treatment might be used for several ends: radiation therapy might be required simply to palliate bone cancer pain, or it may be used to prolong life. Goal-category protocols are commonly found in nursing homes, where they are often known as "Supportive Care," "Comfort Care," or "Routine Terminal Care" protocols (Miles & Ryden, 1985).

Care-category protocols are an attempt to improve communication among medical staff and between medical staff and their patients by clarifying complex treatment plans that selectively use life-sustaining treatments (Committee on Policy, 1983; Meisel et al., 1986). The success of care categories lies in the extent to which this simplified communication is both necessary and successful. Their danger lies in the extent to which the categories fail to accurately communicate treatment intentions. A categorization scheme that accurately conveyed the complex individuality of treatment plans, which was understood by patients, families, and health care providers, and which resulted in accurate treatment-plan implementation would be a potent advance in medical communication.

There is only fragmentary evidence that care categories can achieve this end. Care categories can play a useful role in patient education and counseling (Volicer, Rheaume, Brown, Fabizewski, & Brady, 1986). Treatment categories may simplify William Anderson's choices so that he can choose among a forbidding number of potential treatments. Likewise, goal categories may help Mrs. Swift's family recognize that they are choosing to palliate her as she dies rather than misdirecting their attention to dozens of individual interventions. Care categories can effectively limit medical treatment (Arena, et al., 1980; Mott, 1988). What is missing is the crucial evidence that care categories accurately translate patient preferences into medical treatment.

Treatment categories are difficult to define. Although some patients or physicians might view antibiotics as being in a single category, others might distinguish intravenous antibiotics from oral antibiotics. This problem becomes more difficult as dissimilar therapies are aggregated into a category. Categories that limit transfers to hospitals or intensive care units are especially problematic in that hospitals or intensive care units are distinguished as much by the degree of supervision of care as by interventions or management goals. If the dying Ms. Swift had been admitted to a nursing home while suffering uncontrollable pain or dyspnea, she might instead have preferred the more intensive treatment of a hospital, if assured that the hospital would respect her wish to decline life-sustaining care.

Treatment categories may not be sufficiently flexible. Some hospital protocols would use Mr. Anderson's refusal of CPR to place him in a category where desired treatment for a gastric hemorrhage would not be given in an ICU. Proponents of treatment categories are trying to refine protocols to address this problem (Davila, Boisaubin, & Sears, 1986). Several such protocols specifically state that individual treatment decisions should be carefully described in the medical record notwithstanding the use of categorical descriptors (Davila, et al., 1986; Meisel, 1986). When categories are constructed by protocol drafters, the patient's ability to autonomously define his or her overall treatment plan may be abridged (Lynn, 1986; Uhlmann, Cassel, & McDonald, 1984).

The dichotomization of treatment goals—palliation or prolongation of life—in supportive-care protocols is likewise problematic (Miles & Ryden, 1985). The assumption that a decision to limit life-sustaining treatment entails rejecting prolongation of life is necessary in order to construct separate goal categories. Patients make treatment choices for many reasons including: quality of life, religious convictions, cost, and inconvenience (Tomlinson & Brody, 1988). Many older nursing home residents who, like Mr. Anderson, wish to decline CPR (Wagner, 1984) while continuing to receive less burdensome

TABLE 5.3 Summary of Treatment-Category Protocols[a]

	Highest categories	Intermediate categories	Lowest categories
		HOSPITAL SETTINGS	
Arena, Perlin, & Turnbull (1980)	A. Code. Good long-term prognosis; maximal therapeutic effort.	B. Code. Limited long-term prognosis; effective therapy available; resuscitation/ICU transfer.	C. No-code. Short-term prognosis poor; ordinary therapeutic effort; eligible for ICU only in unusual circumstances.	D. No-code. No further therapy; physical and psychological comfort; no resuscitation; no ICU transfer.
Committee on Policy (1983)	A. All curative and functional maintenance therapies as indicated.	B. Any curative therapy in progress (if any) will be continued until its outcome has been determined; no new curative therapy will be implemented. B1: In the event of cardiopulmonary arrest, the patient is to be resuscitated. B2: DNR.		C. Comfort the patient as he or she is dying.
Clinical Care Committee (1976)	A. Maximal therapeutic effort without reservation.	B. Maximal theraputic effort to be evaluated daily.	C. Selective limitation of therapeutic measures. Not an appropriate candidate for admission to intensive care unit.	D. All indicated therapy can be discontinued. Any measures indicated to ensure maximum comfort of the patient may be continued or instituted.

Davila, Boisaubin, & Sears (1986)	A. Full support, including CPR.	B. Full support, excluding CPR.	C. Modified support excluding CPR.
Executive Committee (1976)	A. All but CPR: May treat vigorously, but if cardiac arrest occurs, no resuscitation is to be attempted, and all treatment is withdrawn.	B. No extraordinary measures: Used for patients with minimal brain function and no hope for improvement. Extraordinary measures include CPR, admission to ICU, parenteral nutrition.	
Meisel, Grenvik, Pinkus, & Snyder (1986)	A. All but cardiac resuscitation.	B. Limited therapy: In general, no additional therapy is initiated except for hygiene comfort; DNR.	C. Comfort measure only; only give nursing and hygienic care and medication appropriate to maintain comfort.

(continued)

TABLE 5.3 (continued)

	Highest categories	Intermediate categories	Lowest categories	
		HOSPITAL SETTINGS (continued)		
Quill, Stankaitis, & Krause (1986)	A. Critical care: Maximal therapeutic effort.	B. Limited critical care: Maximal ordinary and temporary extra-ordinary thera-peutic measures short of CPR; phy-sician must specify which extraordinary measures to include and which to ex-clude in emergency.	C. Conservative care: All ordinary thera-peutic measures, but no CPR or extraordinary measures should be initiated.	D. Comfort-oriented care: Therapeutic efforts are guided by maximizing the patient's comfort regardless of their effect on the disease process.
Volicer (1986)	A. Aggressive diagnostic workup, treatment of coexisting medical conditions, and transfer to an acute care unit if necessary.	B. Same as A., but with DNR.	C. DNR. No transfer to acute care for medical manage-ment of intercurrent life-threatening illnesses.	D. DNR. No transfer to acute care. No workup or antib-iotic treatment of life-threatening infections. Only antipyretics and analgesics are used to ensure patient comfort. E. Supportive care given as defined in D., but eliminate tube feeding when food intake is not possible. Fluids necessary for hydration provided orally if patient is not comatose.

LONG-TERM CARE SETTINGS

	A	B	C	D
Levenson, List, & Zawin (1981)	A. Maximum resuscitative effort within limits of institution. Transfer to hospital if needed. Full-fledged code.	B. Limited effort. Appropriate drugs may be tried. Full-fledged code until a physician says otherwise. If patient survives, transfer to hospital if needed.	C. No resuscitative effort. Do not call a code. Do not send to a hospital.	
Mott & Barker (1988)	A. Maximum care (e.g., hospitalization for surgery and intensive care).	B. Intermediate care (e.g., hospitalization, but avoid surgery or intensive care if possible).	C. Intermediate, less active care (e.g., avoiding hospitalization, but using antibiotics when indicated).	D. Comfort care only (e.g., avoid hospitalizations, antibiotics).

OTHER SETTINGS

	A	B	C	D
Yarrows (1987)	A. Transfer to a hospital, if necessary, and provide any care indicated, including life-support machinery.	B. Transfer to a hospital if medically indicated; however, avoid mechanical ventilation (life support) and CPR if the heart stops.	C. Provide medical care only at the nursing home for the comfort of the patient, including antibiotics, narcotics.	
Callahan (1987)	A. Emergency life-saving interventions (e.g., CPR).	B. Intensive care and advanced life support (e.g., ICUs, respirators).	C. General medical care (e.g., antibiotics, surgery, cancer chemotherapy, artificial hydration, and nutrition).	D. General nursing care for comfort and palliation.

*Definitions in this table are synopses. See cited references for complete definition of categories and their applications.

forms of monitoring or medication, such persons may be rejecting the treatment burden of CPR rather than prolongation of life itself. Ms. Swift is in a
small group of persons who might reject all forms of life-sustaining care
(Brown, Henteleff, Barakat, & Rowe, 1987). Equating the limited use of
life-sustaining treatment with "supportive-care" can be a misleading eu-
phemism that invalidly equates the intent and scope of Mr. Anderson's
treatment plan with that of Ms. Swift's. A published model for such supportive-care plans (Task Force, 1984) has been criticized (Hoyt & Davies, 1984;
Miles, 1984) and withdrawn (Cranford R.E., personal communication, 1987).

The conceptual difficulty with care categories becomes of practical concern when categories empower on-call staff to make momentous decisions
about a patient's care. Decisions about many of the treatments encompassed
by care categories (e.g., hospitalization or antibiotics) are not immediately
obvious from a patient's preference to "avoid machines," "avoid heroics," or
"not be kept alive as a vegetable," and are best evaluated in consultation with
the primary physician or proxies. William Anderson's consent to "supportive care" in order to decline CPR and endotracheal intubation could
endanger his life if on-call staff provide only analgesia for dysuria and fever
because supportive care means to "preserve comfort, hygiene and dignity"
without prolonging life (Miles & Ryden, 1985).

Care categories, despite their difficulties, may have a limited usefulness in
the complex construction of treatment plans. They may offer a useful framework for communicating with patients, for helping to clarify treatment goals
or the relationships between various treatment decisions (Volicer, 1986).
Health care providers might employ *several* care-category schemes depending
on whether the treatment issues devolved on a fundamental shift of treatment goals or a more restricted limitation of treatment burdens. As decision
makers develop a clearer understanding of the treatment plan choices, individualized treatment plan should be constructed in the orders and notes of
the medical record. Care-category designations (e.g., "Supportive Care Only"
or "Class C") should not be used as medical orders or as nursing plans in lieu
of individualized treatment orders (Hoyt & Davies, 1986). Directives to on-
call personnel should be specific and should not authorize on-call personnel
to make discretionary life or death decisions without consulting the primary
physician.

Treatment-Plan Protocols

Treatment-plan protocols allow for individualized treatment plans in a
manner analogous to the usual medical orders. Some offer specific menus
of life-sustaining treatment orders, from which physicians can indicate
their preferences (see Appendix I—University Hospitals of Cleveland).

Others do not even propose such lists of treatments, but instead simply define critical terms (like DNR) for communication with on-call staff (Minnesota Hospital Association, 1986), and describe a procedural framework for implementing treatment plans that withhold or selectively employ life-sustaining treatments.

Treatment-plan protocols attempt to accommodate the complex individuality of Mary Swift's, William Anderson's, or Thomas Johnson's treatment preferences. They are more comprehensive than DNR protocols and avoid the "one size fits all" problem of care categories. These protocols point to the emergence of a new section of the medical record that summarizes the patient's management goals, treatment philosophy, and critical treatment decisions. Forerunners of this type of record or chart section are seen in unpublished nursing home protocols and in new formats for the front page of hospital medical records (Office of Technology Assessment, 1988, p. 72).

Treatment-plan protocols are a recent and incompletely debated model. Proponents of care categories might feel that treatment-plan protocols fail to offer staff and patients a way to grasp dauntingly complex clinical decisions, or that it is impractical to address every life-sustaining treatment individually. If, as was suggested earlier, care categories can play a constructive role in facilitating the early stages of the decision-making process, treatment plan protocols might offer a procedural framework for implementing individualized results of these decision-making processes, and in this sense may be the next logical stage in evolving a plan that fully and effectively addresses a particular patient's needs.

CONCLUSION

Health care facility protocols for the elective use of life-sustaining treatments fundamentally refer to the provision of patient care by clinicians. In addressing clinical decision making and treatment-plan implementation, they must be intelligible to clinicians and realistically address clinical situations. Prototype cases can be an excellent framework for the design of protocols and for staff education. Protocols should propose a view of individualized treatment plans that can assist decision makers in addressing the totality of treatment intentions without limiting the flexibility that is required to meet each patient's needs.

With this foundation, we can now explore the content of health care facility protocols. Provisions establishing a moral framework for treatment decisions are discussed in Chapter 6. Provisions to improve clinical decision making are discussed in Chapter 7. Provisions to improve treatment implementation are discussed in Chapter 8.

CHAPTER **6**

Provisions To Endorse Ethical Principles

Before attempting to govern clinical decision making and treatment-plan implementation directly, protocols set an institutional stage for the elective use of life-sustaining treatments. This stage is a statement of how the elective provision of life-sustaining treatment relates to the facility's identity and mission. Four types of endorsements are especially important to protocols addressing the elective use of life-sustaining treatment. The first is the statement that patient autonomy is the proper moral perspective for evaluating medical treatments. The second is the statement that extra vigilance should be maintained with regard to treatment proposals for vulnerable persons. The third is the statement as to how the institution's mission relates to clinical practices concerning the elective use of life sustaining treatments. Finally are presumptions for addressing situations where the moral views of health care staff conflict with a patient's treatment preferences. This chapter considers how health care facilities have made these statements and communicated this identity to staff, to patients, and to the community.

To be credible, a statement of institutional presumptions for care should be backed by a commitment of institutional resources. An administration that is committed to "the highest ethical standards of decision making" should be willing to allocate staff time for ethics committees and staff training. It should also provide material and administrative support for the incorporation of advance directives into treatment plans and so forth. Mission statements should be not be platitudes. A commitment to "quality health care" goes without saying unless a facility defines its special view of the meaning of that concept.

ENHANCING PATIENT AUTONOMY

Many protocols explicitly affirm the fundamental moral and legal importance of patient autonomy regarding decisions about life-sustaining treatments (Halligan & Hamel, 1985; Hoyt & Davies, 1986; Meisel et al., 1986; Minnesota Hospital Association, 1986; Rabkin et al., 1976; Uhlmann et al., 1987). Thus, one protocol says, "If the patient is competent, he or she has the clear right to refuse any treatment (including resuscitation) even if the consequences of such refusal may be death" (Committee on Policy, 1983, p. 321). Others are more philosophical, "Decisions to forgo life-sustaining treatment are based . . . in the legal and moral right to self determination, that is a person's right to form, revise over time, and pursue his or her own plan of life. . . ." (Halligan & Hamel, 1985, p. 28).

The affirmation of the principle of autonomy is useful in several ways. It conveys to patients and staff the administration's willingness to honor the expressed preferences of patients like William Anderson, Walter Jones, and Susan Swift. It is a useful reference point for designing procedures to promote good decision making, such as the distribution of advance directives (see Chapter 7). It may help staff who consult the protocol for help with unanticipated problems. Though few facilities may anticipate Walter Jones's preference for an unrelated proxy to represent his wishes, respect for autonomy suggests that his request has moral weight. Or, if a protocol limits DNR orders to terminally ill patients (a common error, discussed in Chapter 7), support for autonomy might be invoked to support Mr. Anderson's request to forego resuscitation even though he is not terminally ill. Finally, patients who are aware of institutional support for their treatment preferences may be more inclined to participate in prospective treatment planning. Some states and professional associations have proposed that patient bill of rights that support patient autonomy be posted in patient care areas as a way to empower patients (American Hospital Association, 1973; State of Minnesota, 1974).

PROTECTING VULNERABLE PATIENTS

Protocols address the facility's responsibility to advance the interests of vulnerable patients in several ways. Some state the equal value of the lives of disabled, indigent, or stigmatized persons (Hoyt & Davies, 1986). Some use the language of antidiscrimination (Minnesota Hospital Association, 1986). Some use human rights language: "The life of a person with mental or physical disabilities has the same intrinsic value as that of a person described as normal or healthy. . . . Denial of essential, life maintaining care and life-enhancing care because of mental or physical disabilities is a violation of basic civil and human rights" (Hoyt & Davies, 1986, p. 369).

The vulnerability of patients is especially problematic to the extent to which the institutional milieu or the prejudices of health care providers endangers patients. Patients such as William Anderson, who are able to speak for themselves, are vulnerable mainly to the degree that providers do not establish procedures to accurately incorporate their preferences into treatment plans. In his case, the affirmation of respect for patient autonomy can help empower him. Patients with unusual requests, such as Walter Jones' choice of an unrelated proxy, are vulnerable in that their preferences may be rejected as being too unusual, administratively cumbersome, or because the staff or administration have mistakenly interpreted the law. To the extent that a protocol is able to establish and listen to ethics experts, such vulnerability for patients who can speak on their own behalf can be ameliorated. Rita Jackson is vulnerable in other ways. Prejudicial views about her quality of life might lead health care staff to withhold life-sustaining care (Pearlman & Uhlmann, 1988). Public guardians might subordinate her unique, personal situation to general rules, and refuse to authorize any planning to address the elective use of aggressive life-sustaining treatment. Addressing the vulnerability of Ms. Jackson requires a multifaceted approach which is discussed in Chapter 7.

PROMOTING INSTITUTIONAL MISSION

Evaluation of the use of life-sustaining treatment is an inherently moral act that relates to the central purpose of any health care facility. Some facilities explicitly affirm a benevolent presumption in favor of life-sustaining care. One protocol says "It is the policy of [this hospital] to provide high quality medical care . . . with the objective of sustaining life and practicing in conformance with . . . ethical and medical standards" (Meisel et al., 1986, p. 243). This kind of statement can serve as a foundation for standing orders for aggressive life-sustaining care, like CPR, in medical emergencies where the patient preferences are unknown. It may also support *minimal care standards* incorporating treatments, such as nourishment, which may never be withheld (Koop & Grant, 1986).

Some facilities have specific medical missions that affect the use of life-sustaining treatments. Hospice programs have a view of end of life care that may exclude the provision of therapies like chemotherapy or CPR (Gardner, 1985; Saunders, 1977). A cancer research center has published a protocol that discusses its treatment and respect for cancer patients which recognizes that cancer "may justify but not require heroic measures" (Van Eys et al., 1986, p. 117).

Sectarian facilities, such as Dr. Ruth Steinberg's Shalom Home, are voluntarily associated with communities that have moral views that may address the elective use of life-sustaining treatments or minimal care duties. Such facilities often state a theological perspective on treatment decisions: "We believe that human life is a gift to be treasured, for it is a sharing in the very spirit of God . . . With this policy and all the accompanying guidelines, we affirm our intentions to protect the rights of human life in moments of illness, suffering and death and reaffirm our opposition to euthanasia" (St. Joseph's Hospital, 1984d, p. 365).

Because patients have a nearly unrestricted right to direct their health care, the degree to which a facility with a explicit mission can decline to perform an objectionable treatment proposal is unclear. Health care facility protocols that are created and adopted to answer and refuse a patient's preference to decline such care will probably have little standing. Court decisions suggest that patients may presume that the facility has promised to honor all legal treatment preferences within the technical expertise of the providers (In re Bouvia, 1986; In re Jobes, 1987; Bartling v. Superior Court, 1984; In re Raquenna, 1986). Health care facility missions might have legal standing if the treatment view is grounded in a broader philosophy of care and institutional commitments and if the patient is informed of the facility's mission and its implications for medical treatment as they are admitted to the facility. If an informed patient understands and accepts the terms of a Shalom Home mission statement on elective nourishment at admission, the facility might be able to discharge a patient who subsequently requests a course of treatment that is contrary to the mission. Such a person would of course retain the right to pursue preferred treatments at a different facility.

ACCOMMODATING MORAL VIEWS OF STAFF

The importance of institutional support for allowing health care staff to exempt themselves from treatment plans to which they object is increasingly recognized (American Hospital Association, 1985; Hastings Center, 1987; Meisel et al., 1986; Minnesota Hospital Association, 1986; Uhlmann et al., 1987). These provisions support the mutually voluntary treatment relationship between patients and health care staff (Hastings Center, 1987; President's Commission, 1982). These provisions are analogous to "conscience clauses" by which hospitals have exempted objecting physicians or nurses from participating in abortions. One protocol reads, "health care professionals . . . may decline to provide a particular option because that choice would violate their conscience or professional judgement. In doing this, the patient may not be abandoned" (Halligan & Hamel, 1985, p. 28).

These provisions serve two purposes. They encourage health care staff to develop and hold moral views of health care. Support for the moral integrity of health care providers is an important safeguard for the quality of patient care. Thus, Shalom Home might support Dr. Steinberg's choice to excuse herself from certain treatment plans even if the facility did not find the treatment proposal to be objectionable. Second, these protocols can be used as a way to promote patient autonomy by intervening when a physician refuses to incorporate a patient's preferences into a treatment plan. Thus, if William Anderson's physician feels that it is wrong to withhold CPR from this non-terminally ill man, the physician should be excused from this patient's care. When such provisions are invoked, clinical supervisors should assist in transferring the patient to the care of another provider (usually within the facility) who does not object to the patient's request.

Although exempting objecting staff from certain treatment plans can serve patient and staff needs in exceptional circumstances, it is still disruptive to patient care and to the operation of the facility. Physicians, nurses, or other personnel should be familiarized with the range of health care options that may be anticipated within the facility. Staff whose views fundamentally and frequently diverge from patient's treatment plans and the institution's mission might be counseled to seek employment in a facility where health care will be more compatible with their preferences.

CONCLUSION

Protocols can articulate institutional assumptions for the provision or discontinuation of life-sustaining treatments. This framework should support patient autonomy, vigilance for the interests of vulnerable patients, accomodate strong staff objections to certain treatment proposals, and articulate the facility's mission with regard to the elective provision of life-sustaining treatment. Once this institutional framework is established, the protocol can address the individual treatment-plan decision making and treatment-plan implementation.

CHAPTER 7

Provisions for Good Decision Making

This chapter examines ways that facilities have designed protocols to improve the process of clinical decision making. Decision-making protocols vary greatly in scope and format. Some address only decisions to withhold CPR; newer protocols address a variety of treatment issues. Some propose ethical principles but do not propose procedures to improve the decision-making encounter with patients or families (Halligan & Hamel, 1985; Van Eys et al., 1986). Some emphasize the role of health professional's compassion, respect for life, and beneficence in decision making (Van Eys et al., 1986); others emphasize a patients' rights view of decision making (American Hospital Association, 1973; Hoyt and Davies, 1986; State of Minnesota, 1974).

Decision-making protocols are usually written as guidelines; treatment planning is an individualized process that is not easily confined to the rigid dictates of the policy voice. Thus, protocols do not as a rule propose outcomes for given clinical situations; Mr. Anderson's or Mr. Jones' views may differ from those of other similarly situated patients with a different view of medical care. Simplified outlines of approaches to clinical decision making may be found in medical periodicals (Perkins, 1986; Ruark & Raffin, 1988; Wanzer et al., 1984) and clinical handbooks (see also Appendix V).

We will focus on five aspects of the application of protocols to clinical decision making. Protocols often suggest ways to address decision making for patients who are able to participate in treatment planning, like Mr. Jones or Mr. Anderson. Many protocols address treatment planning for the common situation of patients who are unable to express treatment preferences or who are otherwise vulnerable, like Ms. Jackson or Ms. Swift. Some suggest procedures to assist staff or patients in resolving controversial or disputed treatment proposals. A few protocols propose a role for medical criteria in delimiting the scope of decisions to withhold life-sustaining treatment. Finally, new financial constraints or conflicts are a special problem that might be addressed by administrative protocols.

PATIENTS WITH DECISIONAL CAPACITY

To support patient autonomy, health facility protocols may propose that staff who care for patients like William Anderson or Walter Jones routinely initiate treatment planning for the elective use of life-sustaining treatments. The purpose of advance planning is to give patients time for careful and unpressured reflection on treatment issues at a time when they are best able to participate in treatment decisions. A patient's capacity for thoughtful decision making may be impaired or even absent during medical emergencies. For persons like Mr. Anderson, facilities should foster a process of treatment planning that creates an advance directive for the use of life-sustaining treatments and designates a surrogate to speak on his behalf in the event he is unable to speak for himself (Beth Israel, 1983; Committee on Policy, 1983; Meisel et al., 1986; Uhlmann et al., 1987).

Protocols may make health care staff responsible for initiating this planning and creating a climate in which Mr. Anderson would feel comfortable discussing his treatment preferences (Hastings Center, 1987; Schneiderman & Arras, 1985). Hospitals usually delegate this responsibility to physicians (Halligan & Hamel, 1985; Meisel et al., 1986; Miles et al., 1982). Nursing homes may propose a greater treatment-planning role by nurses or social workers, reflecting the greater prominence of nursing care plans in treatment planning (Besdine, 1983; Miles & Ryden, 1985; President's Commission, 1983). Some have proposed that nurses or social workers conduct initial planning so that patients are knowledgeable before detailed discussions with a physician (Hastings Center, 1987). Some facilities, assigning primary responsibility for treatment planning to physicians, ask nurses to record conversations in which patients express preferences and inform the physician of these conversations (Miles & Moldow, 1984; Read, 1983). This process would solicit the views of persons like Susan Swift who expressed treatment wishes to nurses and family, rather than to her physician (Committee on Policy, 1983).

Some protocols structure a treatment planning encounter at admission. Some nursing homes, for example, routinely initiate treatment planning with all newly admitted residents or their families (Yarrows, 1987). Some hospitals have ICU physicians routinely address possible limits to the use of life-sustaining therapies for all ICU patients (Clinical Care Committee, 1976). Ms. Swift is critically ill and dying of a long illness; it is important and urgent to establish an agreement to limit resuscitation to avoid subjecting her to major invasive therapy. On the other hand, her new physician does not know her or her family. Because advance treatment planning has not been done, a provisional plan to correct dehydration and anemia may well be appropriate, while a treatment plan for the comprehensive use of life-sustaining therapies is discussed with the family.

There are several drawbacks to using admission conferences for treatment planning. Crucial diagnostic or prognostic information may not be available. Newly admitted patients are often ill and under considerable stress. Older patients may have deliriums that diminish their ability to participate in decision making. Patients and families are often not well acquainted with health care staff. Raising this issue may reinforce fears that the patient is going to die or that the provider is planning to abandon the patient in an hour of need (Levenson & List, 1981). Such fears might lead patients or families to express treatment preferences, such as "Do everything!" or "No machines!" that they might reconsider on more careful reflection. The overcrowded admission agenda of acute medical needs and bureaucratic procedures may not accommodate treatment planning. On balance, admission to a facility can be a good time to initiate treatment planning but is rarely an appropriate time to finalize treatment intentions, especially when the patient, family, and medical situation are not well known.

Patient educational materials can be distributed to improve patients' or families' abilities to participate in the treatment-planning process. Some protocols call for the distribution of informational packets with advance directives for treatment preferences or proxy designations (Committee on Policy, 1983; Hastings Center, 1987; Hoyt & Davies, 1986; Los Angeles County Department of Health Services, 1983; McPhail et al, 1981; Mt. Sinai Hospital, 1984; Northwestern Memorial Hospital, 1982; Smith & Wigton, 1987; Stephens, 1986; Uhlmann, et al., 1987; Yarrows, 1987). Some facilities distribute summaries of their protocols (Meisel et al., 1986). During the design process, informational pamphlets should be reviewed by patients or families of patients to ensure that they are comprehensible. The opportunity for knowledgeable counseling should be offered whenever such material is distributed. As discussed in Chapter 5, some facilities introduce care categories as a way to inform patients of the range of options (Volicer, 1986). Patient support groups to discuss such issues have also been proposed (Hoyt & Davies, 1986).

Facilities are increasingly encouraged to ask patients to designate surrogate decision makers. These designated surrogates are presumably more likely than are routinely selected closest kin to be able to speak about the patient's recent preferences and values. Decisionally capable patients, like Mr. Jones, who wish to name an unrelated surrogate, should be encouraged to use a durable power of attorney in view of the customary deference to family (Steinbrook & Lo, 1986). Even though Mr. Anderson's preferences seem clear, he should be encouraged to appoint a proxy as a part of creating a treatment plan so that his preferences might be interpreted as he would wish even though family are available. Facilities should not assume that the family who brings the patient to the facility is the appropriate surrogate.

A few facilities allow physicians to not discuss withholding life-sustaining treatments with the patient if the physician believes that the discussion would harm the patient, not be in the patient's best interest, or if the patient wishes not to be involved in these discussions (Beth Israel Hospital, 1983; Miles & Moldow, 1983). There is only anecdotal support for the "harmfulness" of these discussions. Patients from certain cultural backgrounds may not expect to discuss the elective use of life-sustaining treatment, and certain patients in well-established physician–patient relationships may delegate these decisions to the physician's judgment (Presidents Commission, 1982). In most settings "therapeutic privilege" is probably a rationalization to support the physician's own difficulty in discussing these issues; one protocol admonishes clinicians not to withhold discussions simply because they are unpleasant or upset[ing] (Uhlmann, et al., 1987, Meisel, et al., 1986). Another protocol points out that patients are able to handle increasing amounts of information over time and that information might be revealed gradually in a manner that the physician documents in the medical record (Meisel et al., 1986). Although ethicists are reluctant to support therapeutic privilege, clinicians and ethicists agree that it is wrong to discuss—as if they are elective—the use of futile therapies that will have no effect (Blackhall, 1987), though in such cases the patient or surrogate should still be informed of the positive goals of management and of the unavailability of effective therapies. Protocols that allow for therapeutic privilege usually emphasize that the patient's surrogates must be fully informed participants in treatment decisions when the patient is not.

PATIENTS WITHOUT DECISIONAL CAPACITY

Many patients lack the ability to make decisions about life-sustaining treatments. Some, like William Anderson or Walter Jones, will have planned for this eventuality and communicated treatment or surrogate preferences before losing the ability to express their preferences. Some, like Susan Swift, had strong preferences but did not incorporate them into a treatment plan. Others, like Rita Jackson, lack decisional capacity and are not known to have previously stated treatment preferences; they present a very difficult treatment planning problem. Patients, professional staff, and health care facilities share the responsibility for diminishing the number of such persons by involving patients in advance treatment planning. This section focuses only on an administrative framework for addressing the needs of decisionally incapable patients; substantive discussion of decision making for incapable patients may be found in the references suggested in Appendix V.

Decisional capacity is a critical and disputed concept for planning for the elective use of life-sustaining treatments. The conclusion that Rita Jackson lacks decisional capacity means that she will be unable to fully and directly participate in treatment decisions, and implies a need to empower others to speak as to her preferences and on her behalf. There are legal and clinical definitions of decisional capacity. Incompetence is the conclusion of a judicial procedure that a person is unable to manage some or all of their affairs. Decision-making capacity is a clinical assessment that one possess values and goals, and is able to communicate, understand information and insightfully make choices in light of clinical realities and values (Annas, 1986; Hastings Center, 1987; President's Commission, 1982). There are no simple clinical criteria or tests for measuring decision-making capacity. Protocols often use *competent* or *incompetent* as synonyms for having or not having decision-making capacity.

Reflecting the imprecision of the clinical assessment of decisional capacity, it is not surprising that protocols and models handle this determination in a variety of ways. Some merely note the significance of this assessment to treatment planning and do not define it (McPhail et al., 1981). Others assign the assessment of decisional capacity to the attending physician (Meisel et al., 1986; President's Commission, 1982; Halligan & Hamel, 1985) or a consulting psychiatrist (Beth Israel, 1983). Some protocols list groups of persons who are incapacitated by definition (e.g., unemancipated minors, prisoners, persons under legal guardianships by court order).

More recent versions define decisional capacity (American Health Care Association, 1981; Committee on Policy for DNR Decisions, 1983; Halligan & Hamel, 1985; Hastings Center, 1987; University of Wisconsin, 1983). One protocol definition reads as follows: "a patient who is conscious, able to understand the nature and severity of his or her illness, and the relative risks and alternatives, and able to make informed and deliberate choices about the treatment and illness" (Beth Israel, 1983, p. 502). Some protocols emphasize that decisional capacity is a task-specific, rather than holistic conclusion, for example: "Patients lacking full decision making capacity should be consulted to the degree feasible. Although a patient's memory may be impaired, he or she may understand the ramifications of certain decisions" (Uhlmann et al., 1987, p. 880). Rita Jackson's warm enthusiasm for a frequent visitor might be taken as an affirmation of trust that would justify bringing that person into the decision-making process.

Protocols describe a variety of procedural approaches for treatment planning for patients who are decisionally incapable. Many facilities promote advance treatment planning as for decisionally capable patients. This process should begin in advance of medical crises so that surrogate decision makers may be fully empowered and so that important treatment decisions may be carefully considered rather than made on the spur of the moment (Hilfiker, 1983). Some protocols require treatment planning conferences with physicians, nurses, social workers, and family members (Beth Israel, 1983; McPhail, et al., 1981; Volicer, et al., 1986). Health professionals should seek out family or close friends with an intimate, loving knowledge of such persons. Such conferences can be forums for interdisciplinary communication in which Mrs. Swift's earlier conversations with nurses and family can be discovered. Some protocols state that the facility will honor previously expressed treatment preferences even if a patient later loses decision-making capacity (Uhlmann, et al., 1987). Thus, a critical part of treatment planning is to seek to discover such treatment preferences or relevant past values. Some protocols specifically propose the standard of substituted judgment for decisionally incapable persons: "Decisions made by others on the patient's behalf, should replicate the ones patients would make if they were capable of doing so" (Halligan & Hamel, 1985, p. 29; Miles & Moldow, 1983). However, an unsupported estimate of substituted judgment or best interests, even by well-intentioned caregivers for the incontinent, aphasic, isolated, financially dependent Rita Jackson raises troubling issues about social prejudices and caregiver fatigue or frustration (Anonymous, 1988). Health professionals should be mindful of how prejudicial views of the disabled can adversely affect care and be willing to operate with protections and oversights to protect these vulnerable patients. (See Chapter 2 and below.)

Protocols often call for surrogate decisionmakers for decisionally impaired patients. In most cases, caring family members may fill this role. Health care facilities should be aware that state laws are not uniform with regard to the standing given to family proxies (Areen, 1987). The authority of families may be legally limited by living wills, durable powers of attorney, and guardianship actions. Furthermore, as one protocol puts it, "family . . . do not necessarily have a legal right to impose their wishes or decisions either on a physician or a patient as to the care that is to be rendered" (Northwestern Memorial Hospital, 1982, p. 304). Even without formal assignment, unrelated intimate friends of a patient may be allowed to participate in the decision-making process if they have demonstrated significant, caring knowledge and regard for the patient's preferences and interests (Hastings Center, 1987). Some protocols propose that legally appointed surrogates be used for decisions to forego life-sustaining treatments, especially when family are not available or are divided about the course to be taken (American Health Care Association, 1981; Committee on Policy, 1983; Meisel et al., 1986). Legal guardians may act on a patient's behalf, though they should be challenged if they propose decisions that do not reflect the patient's wishes or interests (LaPuma et al., 1988a). The use of physicians as surrogates, when they have not been specifically appointed by the patient should be discouraged (Uhlmann et al., 1987).

Protocols should try to prevent the misuse of the assessment of decisional capacity to nullify the treatment choices of patients. Walter Jones's preference for CPR despite his physician's reservations should not, by itself, be taken as the inability to make decisions. One protocol states a presumption in favor of the direct participation of patients in treatment decisions unless the basis for the conclusion of decisional incapacity is in the medical record (Meisel, 1986).

VULNERABLE PATIENTS

The fundamental protection for vulnerable persons is an administration and staff that is knowledgeable about and committed to deliberative and accountable treatment planning in collaboration with family, close friends, or community-appointed surrogates, who are actively concerned about the patient's personal welfare. Administrative support for the protection of vulnerable persons begins with staff education. Staff should be sensitive to the needs and perspectives of disabled patients and understand how prejudicial views of the handicapped can adversely affect treatment choices. Staff should be aware of legal requirements for consultation with state ombudsmen or guardian's offices for persons who, like Rita Jackson, are under public guardianship. Staff should be aware of vulnerable adult protection acts, applicable definitions of neglect or abuse (see Chapter 2; also: American Health Care Association, 1981; Hoyt & Davies, 1986; In re Jobes, 1986; Meilander, 1986).

Protocols can establish procedures to safeguard decision making for vulnerable persons (Cournos, 1986; Davila, Boisubin, & Sears, 1986; Koop & Grant, 1986; Paris, 1982). The American Health Care Association (1981) proposes that the degree of procedural safeguards should vary depending on the seriousness of the outcome of the decision. Thus major safeguards would be needed for decisions to withhold life-prolonging therapy from patients without decision-making capacity (Cournos, 1986; Uhlmann et al., 1987). One major safeguard is the use of independent surrogates or advocates to review treatment decisions for impaired persons. Another protection is oversight boards to review decisions for vulnerable patients. Such bodies might include ethics, prognosis, or human rights committees (Cranford & Doudera, 1984; Hoyt & Davies, 1986), or special administrative oversight (Beth Israel Hospital, 1983) to audit cases where decisions to limit treatment have been reached.

Procedures to protect vulnerable persons, such as Rita Jackson, should not be so complex or universally applied as to effectively prevent William Anderson from directing his care. In most cases, there is no need to require that Mr. Anderson's treatment plan be reviewed by a state ombudsman or ethics committee. On the other hand, the simple procedures by which Mr. Anderson's physician writes a DNR order should not be universally applied in a manner that precludes oversight of such orders for isolated, decisionally incapable patients, like Ms. Jackson, who might be improperly induced to refuse or incorrectly construed as refusing life-sustaining treatment (Lynn, 1986; Koop & Grant, 1986).

ASSISTING STAFF WITH DIFFICULT DECISIONS

Protocols should establish ethics committees or consultants to provide expert assistance to their staff in difficult treatment situations (Cranford & Doudera, 1984; Hosford, 1986). Some protocols propose or require ethics committees to address controversial or disputed decisions, like Walter Jones' choice for an unrelated proxy, or as an oversight safeguard for vulnerable patients, like Rita Jackson (Committee on Policy, 1983; Cranford & Doudera, 1984; Halligan & Hamel, 1985; Hastings Center, 1987; In re Jobes, 1987, McPhail et al., 1981; Meisel et al., 1986; Rabkin et al., 1976; Uhlmann et al., 1987). An optimum-care committee of all members of the health care team is used to collate and assemble information, and to clarify treatment issues before acting as an advisor to the attending physician at one hospital (Clinical Care Committee, 1976). The use of interdisciplinary forums in creating protocols and in educating staff is discussed in Chapter 3.

It is not clear that health care facilities can improve decision making or lessen the risk of adverse legal action by routinely requiring consultation with ethics committees. Ethics committees would probably satisfy Joint Commission requirements that facilities have a way to resolve disputed DNR orders (Joint Commission, 1987). The few nursing home protocols or models (American Health Care Association, 1981; Brown BA et al., 1987) that require review of all decisions to limit life-sustaining treatment are the exception (Miles & Moldow, 1984). Courts have been variously disposed toward the necessity or authority of ethics committees that have been proposed by health care facilities to address decisions about life-sustaining treatments (*In re Jobes*, 1987; Wolf, 1986).

Court hearings are a costly, time-consuming, and rarely necessary way to evaluate decisions about life-sustaining treatments (Hastings Center, 1987; Office of Technology Assessment, 1987). Court action is not required to ratify or invoke a durable power of attorney or living will. Because of staff uncertainty about the use of the courts, some facilities' protocols discourage their use or suggest that they mainly be used to naming surrogates for decisionally incapable persons who are not terminally ill (American Health Care Association, 1981; Beth Israel, 1983) or resolving disputes about a patient's competence (Meisel et al., 1986; University of Wisconsin, 1983).

MEDICAL CRITERIA FOR LIMITING TREATMENT

Some protocols propose medical criteria that affect the outcome of decisions about life-sustaining treatment. Some, for example, require that patients be terminally ill as a precondition to permitting a decision to withhold life-sustaining treatment (McPhail et al., 1981; Miles & Moldow, 1984; Miles & Ryden, 1985; Perkins, 1986; St. Joseph's, 1984a; Veterans Administration, 1984). Others propose conditions, such as "serious disability," where treatment *might* be limited (Hastings Center, 1987; Miles & Ryden, 1985; Task Force, 1984).

Some facilities permit orders to withhold life-sustaining treatment without customary oversight (Bar Association of San Francisco, 1983) or consultation with the patient if treatment is futile. Futility should be strictly defined as meaning that the treatment would have no effect. This type of provision might permit a physician to withhold CPR from a dying patient like Susan Swift (Blackhall, 1987). Futility is variously defined in facility protocols as a condition where the patient is irreversibly and terminally ill, and death is imminent, as irreversible coma, and/or as a irreversibly painful dying process (Beth Israel Hospital, 1983; Hoyt & Davies, 1986; McPhail et al., 1981; St. Joseph's, 1984a; University of Wisconsin, 1983). *Futility* is a narrowly defined term that does not exempt the professional from the duty to be honest and forthcoming with the patient and family about the clinical situation and treatment course.

The use of medical criteria in protocols for decisions about life-sustaining treatment is controversial and problematic. Medical criteria are difficult to define: "Terminal" illness is incompletely distinguished from chronic, progressive disease; severe disability is open to various interpretations. Some fear that such criteria may lead health care staff to unjustly withhold life-sustaining treatment from vulnerable, disabled persons like Rita Jackson (see Rothenberg dissent in Hastings Center, 1987; Hoyt & Davies, 1984, 1986). The requirement that a patient be terminally ill before a DNR order is permitted is an arbitrary limit on patient autonomy that may prevent a person like Mr. Anderson, who is not terminally ill, from making a treatment plan (Perkins, 1986). Futility could be misused to override Walter Jones' preference for aggressive care. Though terminally ill, he may well have several years of productive and valued life after emergency care. Despite these objections to the inclusion of medical criteria in protocols, many medical practitioners argue that treatment futility defines a condition that is beyond the scope of patient's autonomy or expertise (Blackhall, 1987). Thus, even protocols with rigorous oversight requirements for vulnerable patients have attempted to define futility (Hoyt & Davies, 1986).

FINANCIAL CONSTRAINTS ON PATIENT CARE

Virtually nothing is written about how protocols might address the effect of financial constraints, profit-sharing arrangements, and capitated reimbursement plans on health providers' recommendations to withhold life-sustaining treatment. The new potential for a conflict of interest between the financial well-being of a facility or its staff and patients' treatment decisions seems to commend institutional positions on this problem (Hastings Center, 1987; Uhlmann et al., 1987). Future protocols should aspire to three ends. (1) They should separate bodies involved in treatment planning from those serving the institution's financial interests. Thus, utilization review committees should not serve as ethics committees to evaluate discontinuing life-sustaining treatments (Hoyt & Davies, 1986; Miles & Ryden, 1985). (2) They should establish procedures to inform patients of providers' financial interests in the use of life-sustaining treatments (Levinson, 1987; Reagan, 1987). Thus, facilities might expand on Health Care Financing Association regulations that require that patients be informed when being transferred from emergency rooms for financial reasons (Health Care Financing Association (HCFA), 1986). Finally, (3) they should establish an advocacy procedure for inpatients whose care is affected by a financial constraint.

CONCLUSION

Protocols for the elective use of life-sustaining treatments should facilitate a good decision-making process. For decisionally capable patients, protocols can foster advance treatment-planning that involves that patient and anticipates the possibility that the patient will, at some future time, not be able to participate in treatment planning. Protocols should also address the common situation of treatment planning for decisionally incapable patients, again providing for advance treatment planning, the use of surrogate decision makers, and the use of substituted judgment. Facilities should try to foster staff sensitivity to patient vulnerability and provide for oversight of critical decisions for patients who are unable to speak on their own behalf. Medical criteria to control decisions about the use of life-sustaining treatment are rarely needed and pose serious definitional problems for protocol design. Protocols should describe mechanisms for resolving disputed treatment decisions. Finally, new protocols should address and seek to minimize the potential financial conflicts of interest that pertain to health care providers who are facilitating decision making regarding the use of life-sustaining treatments.

CHAPTER 8
Provisions for Implementing Decisions

Protocols for the elective use of life-sustaining treatment establish a framework to promote the proper implementation of treatment decisions (Hastings Center, 1987; Kapp, 1987; Office of Technology Assessment, 1987; President's Commission, 1983). Provisions for proper treatment plan implementation should: (1) establish treatment assumptions that safeguard against the unintended withholding of life-sustaining treatment; (2) maintain accountability of staff for decision making and the provision of treatment; (3) provide for accurate communication of treatment intentions; and (4) promote compliance with mandated procedures of outside agencies. Finally, protocols should provide for proper implementation and updating of the protocol itself.

TREATMENT ASSUMPTIONS

Many protocols establish presumptions in favor of treatment to prevent unintended or improperly authorized withholding of life-sustaining treatment. The most common of these is order for emergency life-sustaining care, such as CPR (Committee on Policy, 1983; Davila et al., 1986), which many protocols state quite simply, for example: "failure to write [a DNR] order in the chart will result in the initiation of resuscitative measures" (Northwestern Memorial Hospital, 1983). In facilities with care-category protocols, failure to designate a category means that the patient is assigned to the most aggressive treatment level (Committee on Policy, 1983). For dying patients like Ms. Swift, these standing orders mean that a provisional treatment plan must be constructed soon after admission if a medical emergency is likely to occur very soon. In nursing homes, there is often a standing order to call paramedics for medical emergencies, which thus invokes the standing orders for aggressive treatment of those agencies as well (Levinson et al., 1987).

There is some debate about whether CPR standing orders should be used in nursing homes given the low success rate of this therapy. The possibility that some residents might desire potentially beneficial CPR is a persuasive argument in favor of CPR standing orders so that such persons do not die because of an inadvertently omitted CPR order. Nevertheless, facilities should consider requiring treatment planning for elective use of CPR soon after admission so that patients for whom CPR is not wanted are not subjected to painful and costly overtreatment.

Some protocols default to aggressive treatment if treatment orders are not explicitly clear. Providers who accept do-not-resuscitate orders may not, for example, accept vague or euphemistic directives like "supportive care only," or "in case of emergency page house officer stat." Such providers will instead provide customary aggressive care (Miles & Crimmins, 1985, Committee on Policy, 1983). This would be especially important in interfacility transfers where patients like Mr. Anderson would receive care from the same ambulance service that services several nursing homes, each with their own definition of "limited treatment" or "no-heroics."

Some protocols provide that care categories or orders to withhold care periodically expire if the staff does not restate the continuing appropriateness of withholding treatment. The expiration of orders to limit treatment presumably results in a reassessment of the treatment plan by physicians and patients (Beth Israel, 1983; Davila et al., 1986; Hastings Center, 1987; Somerville Hospital, 1983). For nursing homes, renewal is typically every 1 to 6 months (Miles & Ryden 1985). For hospitals, renewal is every 1 to 7 days, though many allow DNR orders to stand for the duration of the hospitalization (Miles & Moldow, 1984). After orders for DNR or care categories expire, standing orders for full treatment usually apply. If applied to the totality of the treatment plan and not just to orders to withhold resuscitation, this periodic review of the treatment plan would be especially useful for persons like Walter Jones with changing progressive conditions whose treatment preferences are evolving.

Many protocols explicitly create procedures to facilitate revocation of orders to limit treatment when there is reason to believe that the directive no longer reflects the patient's wishes or interests or if the medical facts change. This may be stated quite simply: "The DNR order may be rescinded at any time" (Miles, Cranford, & Schultz, 1983, p. 661). Other facilities establish mechanisms for physicians, nurses, or even family to initiate withdrawal of orders to limit treatment if there is substantial reason to believe that the rationale for withholding care is incorrect (Committee on Policy, 1983; McPhail et al., 1981; Miles & Moldow, 1984; Read, 1983). Such procedures should not empower those who differ with a carefully deliberated treatment plan to overrule the patient's choice when the patient is unable to speak in a medical emergency (Committee on Policy, 1983).

Some protocols define conditions when orders to withhold life-sustaining treatment may be overruled to allow treatment of complications of desired medical treatments. DNR orders may be suspended during and immediately after a desired surgery that necessarily creates physiologic instability or dependence on life-sustaining treatment (Minnesota Hospital Association, 1986). Other policy defines a do-not-intubate order as permitting airway instrumentation for choking or other remediable forms of airway obstruction (Miles & Crimmins, 1985) or permit the emergency treatment of iatrogenic complications (Meisel et al., 1986). Although sound medical rationales can be constructed for these provisions, patients may wish to accept the risks of surgical or medical care and still refuse life-sustaining interventions. Patients should be informed of provisions to override orders to limit treatment (Meisel et al., 1986). If Mr. Anderson is to undergo elective surgery, the implications of this provision for his care in the event of an intraoperative complication should be discussed. Exceptions by mutual agreement of the physician and the patient should be permitted; Ms. Swift should not be placed on a ventilator if she suffers a respiratory arrest as a result of the judicious use of narcotics to relieve her pain.

MAINTAINING ACCOUNTABILITY

Professional accountability is important to each phase of the elective use of life-sustaining treatment: for the decision-making process, for communicating the treatment plan to other health care personnel, and for implementing the treatment plan (Committee on Policy, 1983; Duff, 1979). Specifying professional responsibility ensures that treatment planning and implementation is carried out by those deemed most qualified to do so and also reduces the probability that unauthorized personnel, such as medical students, will improperly improvise treatment decisions. Accountability is served by explicitly assigning responsibility for clinical practices and by establishing a procedural framework that supports or requires that practices are performed by the responsible staff. Chapter 7 discusses professional roles in the decision-making process, this chapter examines professional roles in recording, ordering, and implementing treatment plans.

Physicians are responsible for recording decisions for the elective use of life-sustaining treatments and for initiating implementation of the treatment plan. When several physicians are involved, protocols may suggest way to identify a single physician (Duff, 1979). If responsibility for ordering the elective use of life-sustaining treatments is reassigned, the attending physician should record in the chart how and to whom he or she responsibility has been delegated (St. Joseph's, 1984a). Policies usually require that physicians describe decisions to withhold life-sustaining treatments in the medical record and implement a treatment plan with signed orders in the medical record (Committee on Policy, 1983; Hastings Center, 1987; Joint Commission, 1987; President's Commission, 1983; Rabkin et al., 1976). Teaching hospitals often require attending staff physicians to countersign orders to limit treatment written by physicians-in-training to ensure that senior physicians are aware of and accountable for such decisions (Miles, 1982; Northwestern Memorial Hospital, 1982). The physician need not record "do-not" orders for each conceivable therapy that would not be provided.

Physicians should note the genesis and intent of the treatment plan in the medical record and record the diagnosis, prognosis, patient or proxy wishes, recommendations of the treatment team, treatment objectives, as well as a discussion of key treatment decisions (Bar Association, 1983; Beth Israel 1983; Hastings Center, 1987; Meisel et al., 1986; Rabkin et al., 1976). The note should, however, be explicit and specific enough about treatment issues of immediate concern so that on-call staff do not need to guess about the scope of the treatment plan and can distinguish the plan for Mr. Anderson from that for Ms. Swift. The note should record the basis for the conclusion that a patient is unable to participate in treatment planning, as well as the identity of surrogate decisionmakers and the rationale for selecting them as proxies. Thus, in identifying Mr. Jones' friend as a surrogate decisionmaker despite the availability of family, the note should record that the friend has a close, caring, and recent knowledge of Mr. Jones' illness and treatment preferences and has been selected for that role by Mr. Jones. The note should also include the basis for deciding that treatment is futile when that assessment is affecting the provision of treatment (Hoyt & Davies, 1986; McPhail et al., 1981).

Nurses are sometimes explicitly made responsible for amplifying the record of treatment planning; in addition, they have a major role in the implementation of treatment plans (Miles & Moldow, 1984; Miles & Ryden, 1985). Thus, some facilities require nurses to record discussions they have with patients about such decisions and that physicians are made aware of this information. Nurses are often assigned responsibility for incorporating treatment decisions and medical orders into care plans (see University Hospitals of Cleveland in Appendix I). Some protocols specify implementation duties such as communicating directives to withhold life-sustaining treatment to EMS personnel or relevant off ward personnel.

A few facilities require patients or families to sign advance directives, the medical record, or living wills if life sustaining treatments are to be limited. Although such documents should be encouraged, some persons may not be psychologically capable of committing themselves in writing to a course of action they otherwise might affirm (Rabkin et al., 1976). Yale New Haven Hospital asks patients or families to sign authorizations for DNR orders if the appropriateness of the order is in dispute (Committee on Policy, 1983). Several facilities encourage the inclusion of living wills or durable powers of attorney in a prominent location in the medical record when such documents are available. (Beth Israel, 1983; Hastings Center, 1987; Meisel et al., 1986; Mount Sinai, 1984; Uhlmann et al., 1987). Knowing that their directives will be incorporated into the medical record, families and patients may be encouraged to try to communicate their preferences to health care providers.

COMMUNICATING THE TREATMENT PLAN

Protocols should establish procedures for communicating treatment plans from decisionmakers to personnel who implement them. This involves intrafacility communication as in the communication between those who participated in the treatment planning for William Anderson, Rita Jackson, or Susan Swift and the night or off-ward staff (such as the x-ray department) who are unfamiliar with the patient but who may play a critical role in implementing the treatment plan. Procedures for interfacility communication are also needed for when acutely ill outpatients, like Mr. Jones, or nursing home patients, like Mr. Anderson, are admitted to the hospital by way of an ambulance service. Interfacility communication is also necessary when inpatients, like Ms. Swift, are transferred from a hospital to a nursing home or hospice program.

Protocol provisions for treatment-plan communications serve two goals. First, they promote accurate treatment-plan implementation so that unwanted treatments are not administered and so that wanted therapies are not withheld. Second, they should provide for continuity of accountability for treatment plans; uninformed persons should not be empowered to make new treatment decisions. Clearly documented treatment plans and accountable decision makers presumably exist before communication of treatment plans is contemplated. Empirical studies of how well protocols communicate treatment plans are reviewed in Chapter 2 and Chapter 5.

Physicians are usually assigned responsibility for informing health care staff of the treatment plan (Beth Israel 1983; Committee on Policy, 1893; Minnesota Medical Association, 1983; Rabkin et al., 1976). Protocols have presumably defined important and often-used treatment directives, such as DNR, do-not-intubate, or care categories (see Chapter 5). Some facilities establish new facesheets or sections of the medical record for facilitating communication of decisions about the use of life-sustaining treatment. Some facilities employ DNR wristbands so that off ward staff can be instantly aware of William Andersons's treatment intentions (Minnesota Hospital Association, 1986). In our opinion, if discrete, such bands can reassure a patient that their preferences will be honored. Some facilities have nurses note DNR orders on ancillary service requisition forms (St. Joseph's, 1984a); others reject this approach because of the danger that such forms might be accidentally misapplied to the wrong patient (Committee on Policy, 1983).

Some protocols address orders to withhold life-sustaining treatment that physicians occasionally give by telephone when they are unable to directly supervise care. Such telephone orders may represent an ad hoc decision rather than a carefully thought out plan. If not grounded in a previous discussion with the patient, the telephone order may not take account of patient preferences. Some protocols address the use of telephoned orders for decisions to limit life-sustaining treatment. Some protocols prohibit them (Meisel et al., 1986). Some protocols require that nurses record in writing their discussion with a physician (St. Joseph's, 1984a). Some provide for the expiration of telephoned orders if the physician does not countersign them within 12 to 24 or 72 hours (Miles & Moldow, 1985; Miles & Ryden, 1985; Northwestern Memorial Hospital, 1983).

Transfer of patients from private homes or long-term care facilities to ambulance services to hospitals or from hospitals to nursing homes involves problematic interfacility communication. During these transfers, patients will often be unable to express treatment preferences and providers will often not know the patient's history or condition. Transfers during acute illness may require immediate treatment decisions with serious and long-lasting consequences including death or prolonged invasive lifesupport. In these situations, protocols establish procedures whereby decision making is undertaken by one set of providers and treatment implementation by another (see section on emergency medical services in Chapter 2).

In providing for inter-facility transfers, protocols should provide for: (1) explicit and mutually understood definitions of treatment directives; and (2) readily accessible, dated, treatment orders that bear the recognized signature of a physician. Nursing home records could have special-treatment-order sheets for communicating special-treatment orders to ambulance personnel. Outpatients, like Mr. Jones, and their surrogates should keep similar advance directives readily available for health care personnel who should in turn be empowered by a protocol to accept and honor them (Death at a New York Hospital, 1985). Living wills rarely communicate sufficient diagnostic or therapeutic information to be useful as treatment orders in a medical emergency (Eisendrath & Jonsen, 1983; Schneiderman & Arras, 1985); specific treatment directives designed for such situations will be needed. Formal durable powers of attorney or guardianship decrees can unambiguously identify a surrogate decision maker to health personnel and thus should be honored. Health facility protocols should be designed to conform to a procedural format negotiated with EMS services (Hastings Center, 1987; Marshall, 1985; Miles & Crimmins, 1985). For this to happen, the routine of interfacility transfers should be anticipated so that interfacility agreements can be negotiated and patient preferences with regard to such transfers can be elicited and incorporated into treatment planning.

Discharge documents should clearly describe treatment planning and may issue directives to cover the use of life-sustaining treatments during the transfer. Physicians should not be allowed to make orders to limit medical treatment beyond the time required to transfer the patient to another health care provider who assumes responsibility for the treatment plan. A physician should be continually responsible for treatment orders, so that desired changes can be made.

COMPLIANCE WITH EXTERNAL AGENCIES

Many state governments have requirements as to the handling of orders to withhold CPR or other life-sustaining treatments electively for institutionalized persons who are under state guardianship or who are without close family. Some protocols identify classes of persons to whom such laws apply, and refer decisions to the facility's lawyer or to the identified government body. Health facility protocols should make it clear that the special restrictions or requirements for persons under the purview of government offices do not necessarily apply to all patients in the facility. Thus, even if a state guardian's office will not authorize a DNR order for a non-terminally ill persons, it does not mean that Mr. Anderson can not have such a request honored.

Protocols should provide for compliance with legal requirements regarding living wills, durable powers of attorney, and other relevant matters (e.g., organ donation or brain death). Despite these regulations, patients will often have their own ways of expressing themselves with a living will. One protocol encourages staff to read the intent of the document, not merely to evaluate how closely it conforms to procedural details (Meisel et al., 1986).

PROTOCOL IMPLEMENTATION

Few protocols describe administrative responsibilities to provide for the proper elective use of life-sustaining treatment (Joint Commission, 1987; Minnesota Hospital Association, 1986). Protocols should make the chief executive officer responsible for oversee the implementation of the administrative structures provided for in the protocol. Various offices within the facility might be assigned responsibility for conducting staff education, providing documents (i.e., advance directives, treatment-plan facesheets) or offices (i.e., legal counsel or ethics committees), overseeing quality-assurance audits, and monitoring the adequacy of the facility's framework for the elective use of life-sustaining treatments. The trustees of Shalom Home might endorse a policy that makes Dr. Steinberg responsible for conducting ongoing inservice training and quality-assurance audits, the rabbi's office responsible for supporting the ethics committee, and the assistant director responsible for seeing that durable power of attorneys are readily available to and properly used by social workers and clinicians. An outline of administrative duties is given in Chapter 2.

Protocols for elective use of life-sustaining treatment should be coordinated with other administrative documents and procedures. They should revoke outdated documents or procedures that they replace. They should inform staff of other protocols that are relevant to the treatment planning or implementation (e.g., for organ donation, the determination of brain death, or decision-making guides for comatose patients). Thus, a protocol might alert staff to cornea-donation procedures in the event that Mr. Anderson wishes to make this gift in the course of his treatment planning.

Finally, protocols should have an expiration date. This date should occasion a review of the ongoing adequacy of the protocol in light of information from new legal and bioethical policy, external agencies' procedures, and internal quality-assurance audits. This review can be similar to, though perhaps not as extensive as, the collaborative process to develop the protocol. Building on experience, this review should reexamine clinical practices and the facility's efforts to improve care by means of protocols, ethics committees, charting systems, and the like. This review should lead to further staff education, protocol changes, or other administrative actions. Anecdotal experience suggests this review should be considered every 1 to 3 years, giving sufficient time to implement, evaluate, and reflect on changes in clinical practices.

CONCLUSION

Protocols establish a procedural framework for ethical, safe, accurate, accountable, and legal patient care after treatment decisions have been properly made. This framework is primarily a system of reliable communication between the providers within and outside the facility who share responsibility for patient care. This system of communication is founded on informed and dedicated leadership that supports ongoing staff training, audits of clinical practices, and continual efforts to improve the quality of patient care.

Afterword

Protocols and Moral Life in Institutions

For every human problem, there is a solution
that is simple, neat, and wrong.*

This is a difficult time to propose public protocols to address ethical issues. We do not have a public consensus on a single set of absolute moral principles (McIntyre, 1979). Our institutions are corporate entities whose conduct and interests seem to transcend those of the people who work in or are served by them. Health facility "ethics" protocols address a changing set of intimate relationships between morally diverse strangers: physicians, nurses, patients and families. Finally, many of the ethical dilemmas pertaining to the use of life-sustaining technologies do not present a clear choice between right and wrong but rather offer tragic, and to some degree unsolvable, questions of how to live when human life is at once precious and mortal.

Health facility protocols present many dangers. There is a danger in the belief that clearly stated principles or procedures can definitively solve

* This observation was attributed by President Carter to H.L. Mencken. It hangs on the wall at the Hastings Institute, from whence Stephen Toulmin recorded it (Toulmin, 1981, p. 31).

individual dilemmas (Toulmin, 1981). The sentiment "There ought to be a law!" will as often need to be balanced with the conclusion that, "But, this case is an exception!" There is a danger that protocols or "bioethics expertise" will undermine individual responsibility and insight. Expert policies and sanctioned "right thinking" can lead to "a loss of confidence in private moral initiative," and an impoverished, though procedurally correct, institutional life (Hoff, 1982, p. 13). In this situation, protocols and procedures can transfer clinical control to well-intentioned but remote persons who lack a nuanced feel for the distinctive feelings and facts of each case. Worse, protocols can paralyze personalized decision making by diffusing responsibility or by preempting healthy debate by administrative edict.

In this climate, protocols for the elective use of life-sustaining treatments can play a constructive albeit circumscribed role in improving health care practices. They can illuminate the diverse responsibilities of health care professionals and institutions. They can stress the legitimacy of moral pluralism on these life-and-death issues, and promote a peaceable tolerance and mutual accommodation of differing views (Englehart, 1987). They can establish a framework to promote patient-centered decision making and accurate, accountable treatment-plan implementation.

Moral life in public institutions arises from the discretionary exercise of personal virtues—integrity, empathy, compassion, and judgment. Public policy has affirmed that choices regarding life-sustaining treatment are not to be dictated by law, courts, or health facility administrators. The best choices are those that are the collaborative product of a dialogue between patients, their loved ones, and the professionals who work with them (Siegler, 1981). Ultimately, the role of protocols is to give permission, to inform, and to facilitate responsible private decisions.

References

LEGAL CITATIONS

Bartling v. Superior Court, 163 Cal. App. 3d 186, 209 Cal. Rptr. 220 (Ct. App. 1984).

Bouvia v. Superior Court (Glenchur), 179 Cal. App. 3d 1127, 225 Cal. Rptr. 297 (Ct. App. 1986), *review denied*, Cal. June 5, 1986).

Brophy v. New England Sinai Hospital, Inc., 398 Mass. 417, 497 N.E. 2d 626 (1986).

In re Conroy, 98 N.J. 321, 486 A.2d 1209 (1985).

Darling v. Charleston Community Memorial Hospital, 33 Ill.2d 326, 211 N.E.2d 253 (1965).

In re Dinnerstein, 6 Mas. App. 466, 380 N.E. 2d 134 (Ct. App. 1978).

In re Hier, 18 Mass. App. 200, 464 N.E. 2d 959 (Ct. App.), *review denied*, 392 Mass. 1102, 465 N.E. 2d 261 (1984).

Hoyt v. St. Mary's Rehabilitation Center, No. 773555 (District Ct. Hennepin County, Minn. February 13, 1981), reversed on other grounds *sub nom.* State v. Hoyt, 304 N.W.2d 884 (Minn. 1981).

In re Jobes, 108 NJ. 394, 529 A. 2d 434 (1987).

In re Quinlan, 70 NJ. 10, 355 A.2d 647, *cert. denied sub nom. Garger v. New Jersey*, 429 U.S. 922 (1976), *overruled inpart, In re* Conroy, 98 N.J. 321, 486 A.2d 1209 (1985).

In re Raquenna, 213 N.J. Super. 443, 517, A.2d 869 (Super Ct. App. Div. 1986) (per curiam).

REFERENCES

Abrams FR. Withholding treatment when death is not imminent. Geriatrics 1987; 42(May):77-84.

Abramson NS, Meisel A, Safar P. Deferred consent: A new approach for resuscitation research on comatose patients. JAMA 1986; 255(18):2466-2471.

Ad Hoc Committee of the Harvard Medical School to Examine the Definition of Brain Death. A definition of irreversible coma. JAMA 1968; 205:337-340.

Ad Hoc Committee on Cardiopulmonary Resuscitation of the Division of Medical Sciences National Academy of Sciences—National Research Council. Cardiopulmonary resuscitation. JAMA 1966; 198:373-379.

Ad Hoc Committee on Nursing Home Care of the King County Medical Society. Principles for determining code status of patients in nursing homes. King County Medical Society Bulletin 1985; 64:13-16.

Allen EV, Miles SH. Ethics committees in Minnesota hospitals. Minn Med 1987; 70:77-80.

American College of Emergency Physicians. Medical, moral, legal, and ethical aspects of resuscitation for patients who will have minimal ability to function or ultimately survive. Ann Emerg Med 1985; 14(9):919-926.

American College of Physicians, Ad Hoc Committee on Medical Ethics. Ethics Manual. Philadelphia: American College of Physicians, 1984.

American Health Care Association. AHCA Policy Paper: Patient's rights. Am Health Care Assoc J 1981; 7(5):55-60.

American Heart Association, National Academy of Sciences/National Research Council. Standards and guidelines for cardiopulmonary resuscitation (CPR) and emergency cardiac care (ECC). JAMA 1980; 244:457.

American Hospital Association. Statement on a patient's bill of rights. Hospitals 1973; 47(4):41.

American Hospital Association. Policy and statement: The patient's choice of treatment options. Chicago: American Hospital Association, 1984.

American Hospital Association. Guidelines on establishment of hospital committees to consider biomedical ethical issues. Chicago: American Hospital Association, 1984.

American Hospital Association. Values in conflict: Resolving ethical issues in hospital care. Chicago: American Hospital Association, 1985.

American Medical Association, Council on Ethical and Judicial Affairs. Statement on withholding or withdrawing life-prolonging treatment. Current Opinions of the Council on Ethical and Judicial Affairs of the American Medical Association. Chicago: American Medical Association, 1986.

American Nurses' Association Committee on Ethics. Guidelines for nurse participation and leadership in institutional ethical review processes. Kansas City, MO: American Nurses Association, 1984.

Angell M. The quality of mercy. N Engl J Med 1982; 306(2):98-99.

Angell M. Respecting the autonomy of competent patients. N Engl J Med 1984; 310(17):1115-1116.

Annas GJ. CPR: When the beat should stop. *Hastings Cent Rep* 1982; *12*(5)30-31.

Annas GJ. When procedures limit rights: From Quinlan to Conroy. *Hastings Cent Rep* 1985; *15*(2):24-27.

Annas GJ, Glantz LH. Withholding and withdrawing of life-sustaining treatment for elderly incompetent patients: A review of court decision and legislative approaches. Washington, DC: Office of Technology Assessment, U.S. Congress, 1986:

Annas GJ. Transferring the ethical hot potato. *Hastings Cent Rep* 1987; *17*:20-21.

Anonymous. It's over, Debbie. *JAMA* 1988; *259*(2):272.

Areen GJ. The legal status of consent obtained from families of adult patients to withhold or withdraw treatment. *JAMA* 1987; *258*(2):229-235.

Arena FP, Perlin M, Turnbull AD. Initial experience with a 'code-no code' resuscitation system in cancer patients. *Crit Care Med* 1980; *8*(12):733-735.

Arnold RM. University of Pennsylvania, Philadelphia, PA, personal communication, 1987.

Bader D. Senior Associate for Clinical Ethics, Catholic Health Association of the United States, St. Louis, MO, personal communication, 1988.

Bar Association of San Francisco and the San Francisco Medical Society. Policy statement on orders against resuscitation. In President's Commission for the Study of Ethical Problems in Medicine and Biomedical and Behavioral Research, ed. *Deciding to Forego Life-Sustaining Treatment.* Washington, DC: U.S. Government Printing Office, 1983.

Bardsley & Haslacher, Inc. Awareness and incidence of having a 'living will' in Oregon. Report prepared for Oregon Health Decisions, 1986.

Baskett PJF. The ethics of resuscitation. *Br Med J* 1986; *293*(July 19):189-90.

Bayley C, Cranford RA. Techniques for committee self-education and institution-wide education. In Cranford and Doudera, eds., *Institutional ethics committees and health care decisionmaking.* Ann Arbor, MI: Health Administration Press, 1984.

Bedell SE, Delbanco TL. Choices about cardiopulmonary resuscitation in the hospital: When do physicians talk to their patients? *N Engl J Med* 1984; *310*:1089-1093.

Bedell SE, Delbanco TL, Cook EF, Epstein FH. Survival after cardiopulmonary Resuscitation in the hospital. *N Engl J Med* 1983; *309*(10):569-576.

Bedell SE, Pelle D, Maher PL, Cleary PD. Do-not-resuscitate orders for critically ill patients in the hospital: How are they used and what is their impact? *JAMA* 1986; *256*(2):233-237.

Berger S. Consultant, National Citizens' Coalition for Nursing Home Reform, Washington, DC, personal communication, 1988.

Bertolet MM, Goldsmith LS, eds. *Hospital liability: Law and tactics,* 4th ed., Chicago: Practicing Law Institute, 1980.

Berwick DM, Knapp MG. Theory and practice for measuring health care quality. *Health Care Financing Review* 1987; Supp:49-55.

Besdine RW. Decisions to withhold treatment from nursing home residents. *J Am Geriatr Soc* 1983; *31*(10):602-606.

Beth Israel Hospital (Boston, MA). Guidelines: Orders not to resuscitate. In President's Commission for the Study of Ethical Problems in Medicine and Biomedical and Behavioral Research, ed. *Deciding to Forego Life-Sustaining Treatment.* Washington, DC: U.S. Government Printing Office, 1983.

Blackhall LJ. Must we always use CPR? *N Engl J Med* 1987; *317*(20):1281–1285.

Board of Directors, American College of Emergency Physicians. Directors consider council resolutions. *ACEP News* 1986; October 4.

Board of Directors, American College of Emergency Physicians. Policy statements. *ACEP News* 1987; January 2.

Board of Trustees Minnesota Medical Association. Implementation and transfer of limited treatment orders from long term care facilities to emergency service providers. *Minn Med* 1986; *69*:83–85.

Bowen O. Shattuck lecture: What is quality care? *N Engl J Med* 1987; *316*(25):1578–1580.

Braithewaite S, Thomasma DC. New guidelines on foregoing life-sustaining treatment in incompetent patients: An anti-cruelty policy. *Ann Intern Med* 1986; *104*:711–715.

Brenner LH, Gerken EA. Informed consent: Myths and risk management alternatives. *QRB* 1986; December:420–425.

Brett AS, McCullough LB. When patients request specific interventions: Defining the limits of the physician's obligation. *N Engl J Med* 1986; *315*:1347–1351.

Brook RH, davies-Avery A, Greenfield S. Assessing the quality of medical care using outcome measures: An overview of method. *Med Care* 1977; *15*(9-Suppl):1–165.

Brown BA, Miles SH, Aroskar M. The prevalence and design of nursing home ethics committees. *J Am Geriatr Soc* 1987; *35*(11):1028–1033.

Brown JH, Henteleff P, Barakat S, Rowe CJ. Is it normal for terminally ill patients to desire death? *Am J Psychiatry* 1987; *143*(2):208–211.

Brown NK, Thompson DJ. Non-treatment of fever in extended-care facilities. *N Engl J Med* 1979; *300*:1246–1250.

Burmeister R. Blast or boost? *QRB* 1986; December:417–19.

Byrne RP. Deciding for the legally incompetent. In Doudera and Peters, eds., *Legal and ethical aspects of treating critically and terminally ill patients.* Washington, DC: AUPHA Press, 1982.

California Nurses' Association Ethics Committee. *Statement on the nurse's role in withholding and withdrawing life-sustaining treatment,* adopted May 17, 1987.

Callahan D. *Setting limits: Medical goals in an aging society.* New York: Simon & Schuster, 1987.

Campbell-Taylor I, Fisher RH. The clinical case against tube feeding in palliative care of the elderly. *J Am Geriatr Soc* 1987; *35*:1100–1104.

Campion EW, Mulley AG, Goldstein AL. Medical intensive care for the elderly: A study of current use, costs, and outcomes. *JAMA* 1981; *246*(18):2052–2056.

Capron AM. Ironies and tensions in feeding the dying. *Hastings Cent Rep* 1984; October:32–35.

Carlson RW, Devich L, Frank RR. Development of a Comprehensive supportive care team for the hopelessly ill on a university hospital medical service. *JAMA* 1988; *259*(3):378–383.

Carson RA, Siegler M. Does "doing everything" include CPR? *Hastings Cent Rep* 1982; October:27-29.

Cassel CK. Decisions to forgo life-sustaining therapy: The limits of ethics. *Soc Service Rev* 1987; December:552-564.

Cassel CK, Glasser G, Zweibel NR. Institutional mechanisms for ethical decision-making in nursing homes. *Gerontologist* 1986; 26(spec):123A.

Charlson ME, Sax FL, MacKenzie CR, Fields SD, Braham RL, Douglas G. Resuscitation: How do we decide? A prospective study of physicians' preferences and the clinical course of hospitalized patients. *JAMA* 1986; 255(10):1316-1322.

Chernow B, Seeland AD, Snyder R. Orders not to resuscitate: The DNR patient. *Critical Care* 1984; 12(10):922-923.

Chipman C, Adelman R, Sexton G. Criteria for cessation of CPR in the emergency department. *Ann Emerg Med* 1981; 10(1):11-17.

City of Boston Department of Health and Hospitals. Guidelines: Do not resuscitate orders. In President's Commission for the Study of Ethical Problems in Medicine and Biomedical and Behavioral Research, ed. *Deciding to Forego Life-Sustaining Treatment*. Washington, DC: U.S. Government Printing Office, 1983.

Clinical Care Committee of the Massachussetts General Hospital. Optimum care for hopelessly ill patients. *N Engl J Med* 1976; 295:362-364.

Cohen CB. Interdisciplinary consultation on the care of the critically ill and dying: The role of one hospital ethics committee. *Critical Care* 1982; 10(11):776-784.

Cohen E. Civil liability for providing unwanted life support. *BioLaw* 1987; 2(6):U:499-U:502.

Committee on Ethics and Medical-Legal Affairs. Institutional ethics committees: Roles, responsibilities, and benefits for physicians. *Minn Med* 1985; 68:607-612.

Committee on Policy for DNR Decisions, Yale New Haven Hospital. Report on do not resuscitate decisions. *Conn Med* 1983; 47(8):477- 83.

Concern for Dying. *A living will*. New York: Concern for Dying, 1987.

Connery JR. The ethical standards for withholding/withdrawing nutrition and hydration. *Issues in Law and Medicine* 1986; 2(2):87-98.

Cournos F. Orders not to resuscitate and the psychiatric hospital. *Psychiatr Q* 1986; 58(1):24-31.

Cranford RE. Personal communication, 1987.

Cranford RE, Ashley BZ. Ethical and legal aspects of dementia. *Neurol Clin* 1986; 4(2):479-489.

Cranford RE, Doudera AE, eds. *Institutional ethics committees and health care decisionmaking*. Ann Arbor, MI: AUPHA Press, 1984.

Cranford RE, Van Allen EJ. The implications and applications of institutional ethics committees. *Bull Am Coll Sur* 1985; June:19-24.

Crispell KR, Gomez CF. Proper care for the dying: A critical public issue. *J Med Ethics* 1987; 13:74-80.

Curran WJ. Quality of life and treatment decisions: The Canadian law reform report. *N Engl J Med* 1984; 310(5):297-298.

Curran WJ. A further solution to the malpractice problem: Corporate liability and risk management in hospitals. *N Engl J Med* 1984; 304(11):704-705.

Cushing M. "No code" orders: Current developments and the nursing director's role. *J Nurs Adm* 1981; *11*(4):22-29.

Davila F, Boisaubin EV, Sears DA. Patient care categories: An approach to do-not-resuscitate decisions in a public teaching hospital. *Crit Care Med* 1986; *14*(12):1066-1067.

Davis FA. Quality of health care measurement: A research priority. *Health Care Financing Review* 1987; Supp:1-3.

Death At A New York Hospital (with medical and legal commentary). *Law, Medicine, and Health Care* 1985; *13*:267-282.

DeBard ML. Cardiopulmonary resuscitation: Analysis of six years' experience and review of the literature. *Ann Emerg Med* 1981; *10*:408-416.

Deputy Attorney General for Medicaid Fraud Control, Supreme Court of the State of New York, Queens County Criminal Term Grand Jury Report. *Report of the special January third additional 1983 grand jury concerning "do-not-resuscitate" procedures at a certain hospital in Queens County,* 1983.

Detsky AS, Stricker SC, Mulley AG, Thibault GE. Prognosis, survival, and the expenditure of hospital resources for patients in an intensive-care unit. *N Engl J Med* 1981; *305*(12):667-672.

Dille EJ. Hospital resuscitation policy and the right to be informed. *Health Prog* 1986; October:8-9.

Donabedian A. Evaluating the quality of medical care. *Milbank Memorial Fund Quarterly,* 1966;*44*(3):166-206.

Donabedian A. Commentary on some studies of the quality of care. *Health Care Financing Review* 1987; Supp:75-85.

Donnelly WJ. DNR: The case for early retirement. *Arch Intern Med* 1987; *147*(1):37-38.

Dornette WHC. The legal impact on voluntary standards in civil actions against the health care facility. *New York Law School Law Review* 1977; *22*:925-942

Doudera AE, Peters JD. *Legal and ethical aspects of treating critically and terminally ill patients.* Washington, DC: AUPHA Press, 1982.

Duff RS. Guidelines for deciding the care of critically ill or dying patients. *Pediatrics* 1979; *64*(1):17-23.

Dyck A. Ethical apects of care for the dying incompetent. *J Am Geriatr Soc* 1984; *32*(9):661-64.

Eisendrath SJ, Jonsen AR. The living will: Help or hindrance? *JAMA* 1983; *249*:2054-2058.

Emanuel EJ. Should physicians withhold life-sustaining care from patients who are not terminally ill? *Lancet* 1988; January 16:106-108.

Emanuel EJ. What criteria should guide decision makers for incompetent patients? *Lancet* 1988; January 23:170-171.

Ende J, Grodin MA. Do not resuscitate: An issue for the elderly. *J Am Geriatr Soc* 1986; *34*(11):833-834.

Englehardt HT. *The foundations of bioethics.* New York: Oxford University Press, 1986.

Evans AL, Brody BA. The do-not-resuscitate order in teaching hospitals. *JAMA* 1985; *253*(15):2236-2239.

Everitt DE. Cost containment and the elderly: Making financial incentives more explicit. *J Geriatr Psych* 1985; 18:155-175.

Executive Committee of Presbyterian University Hospital. Guidelines for the care of hopeless/moribund patients. In Cyril Weldt Course Handbook Series, ed. *Medical ethics and legal liability.* New York, NY: Practicing Law Institute, 1976.

Farber NJ. Cardiopulmonary resuscitation (CPR): Patient factors and decisionmaking. *Arch Intern Med* 1984; 144:2229-2232.

Flaherty MJ. The nurse and orders not to resuscitate. *Hastings Cent Rep* 1977; 7(4):27-28.

Fletcher J. Medical resistance to the right to die. *J Am Geriatr Soc* 1987; 35:679-682.

Fogel B, Forrow L, Arnold RM. *The decision to limit life support—A medical procedure.* Unpublished, 1988.

Fox JE. Army initiates "do-not-resuscitate" option for terminally ill patients. *U S Medicine* 1985; June 15:1,14.

Fox M, Lipton HL. The decision to perform cardiopulmonary resuscitation. *N Engl J Med* 1983; 309(10):607-608.

Frampton MW, Mayewski RJ. Physicians' and nurses' attitudes toward withholding treatment in a community hospital. *J Gen Intern Med* 1987; 2:394-399.

Freedman B. On the rights of the voiceless. *J Med Phil* 1978; 3(3):196-210.

Freedman B. Five red herrings and an issue: Response to McCormick. *J Med Phil* 1978; 3(3):222-25.

Fried C. Terminating life support: Out of the closet! *N Engl J Med* 1976; 295(7):390-391.

Fusgen I, Summa J-D. How much sense is there in an attempt to resuscitate an aged person? *Gerontology* 1978; 24:37-45.

Gardner K ed. *Quality of care for the terminally ill—An examination of the issues.* Chicago: Joint Commission on Accreditation of Hospitals, 1985.

Gillick M. The ethics of cardiovascular resuscitation: Another look. *Ethics in Science and Medicine* 1980; 7:161-169.

Glantz LH, Swazey JP. Decisions not to treat: The Saikewicz case and its aftermath. *Forum on Medicine* 1979; January:22-32.

Glasser G, Zweibel NR, Cassel CK. The ethics committee in the nursing home: Results of a national survey. *J Am Geriatr Soc* 1988; 36(2):150-156.

Goodin RE. *Protecting the vulnerable: An analysis of our social responsibilities.* Chicago: University of Chicago Press, 1985.

Goodwin JS, Goodwin JM. Second thoughts: CPR. *J Chron Dis* 1985; 38(8):717-719.

Gordon M. *Problems and challenges in formulating and implementing do not resuscitate policies for an institutionalized elderly population.* Presentation at Annual Meeting of the Gerontological Society of America, Washington, DC, November 20, 1987.

Gordon M, Hurowitz E. Cardiopulmonary resuscitation of the elderly. *J Am Geriatr Soc* 1984; 32:930-934.

Graham H, Livesley B. Dying as a diagnosis: Difficulties of communication and management in elderly patients. *Lancet* 1983; September 17:670-672.

Gramelspacher GP, Howell JD, Young MJ. Perceptions of ethical problems by nurses and doctors. *Arch Intern Med* 1986; *146*:577-578.

Grand Jury of the Supreme Court of the State of New York Queens County. DNR Procedures: Purple dots revisited. *Conn Med* 1985; *49*(6):367-376.

Greenlaw J. Orders not to resuscitate: Dilemma for acute care as well as long-term care facilities. *Law, Medicine, and Health Care* 1982; *10*(1):29-31.

Greenlaw J. Where are we going with 'do not resuscitate' policies? *NY State J Med* 1986; *86*:618-620.

Gunasekera NPR, Tiller DJ, Clements LTS-J, Bhattacharya BK. Elderly patients' views on cardiopulmonary resuscitation. *Age Ageing* 1986; *15*:364-368.

Gustafson JM. The voices of moral discourse. Unpublished lecture, University of Chicago, 1988.

Halligan M, Hamel RP. Ethics committee develops supportive care guidelines. *Health Prog* 1985; *60*:26-30.

Harris S. General Counsel, American Health Care Association, Washington, DC, personal communication, October 15, 1987.

Hastings Center. *Guidelines on the termination of life-sustaining treatment and the care of the dying.* Briarcliff Manor, NY: Hastings Center, 1987.

Haynes BE, Niemann JT. Letting go: DNR orders in pre-hospital care. *JAMA* 1985; *254*(4):532-533.

Health Care Financing Administration (HCFA), Health Standards and Quality Bureau, U.S. Department of Health, Education, and Welfare. *Interpretive guidelines and survey procedures for the application of the conditions of participation for skilled nursing facilities.* Washington, DC: U.S. Government Printing Office, 1979.

Health Care Financing Administration (HCFA), U.S. Department of Health and Human Services. *Medicare/Medicaid skilled nursing facility and intermediate facility survey report (Parts A & B).* Washington, DC: U.S. Government Printing Office, 1985.

Health Care Financing Administration, U.S. Department of Health and Human Services. *Medicare/Medicaid Hospital Survey Report, Form HCFA-1537 (4-86).* Washington, DC: U.S. Govt. Printing Office, 1986.

Hershey CO. Cardiopulmonary resuscitation in general hospital wards. Time to reevaluate. *Int J Cardiol* 1982; *1*(5/6):454-58.

Hilfiker D. Allowing the debilitated to die: Facing our ethical choices. *N Engl J Med* 1983; *308*(12):716-719.

Hilman AL. Financial incentives for physicians in HMO's: Is there a conflict of interest? *N Engl J Med* 1987; *317*(27):1743-1748.

Hoff C. When public policy replaces private ethics. *Hastings Cent Rep* 1982; August:13-14.

Hosford B. *Bioethics committees.* Rockville, MD: Aspen Systems, 1986.

Hospital Council of Southern California. *Life support survey.* Filing code GI-171, Los Angeles, June 26, 1984.

Hoyt J. Chairperson, Nursing Home Action Group, Minneapolis, MN, personal communication, February 22, 1988.

Hoyt JD, Davies JM. A response to the task force on supportive care. *Law, Medicine, and Health Care* 1984; 12(3):103-105.

Hoyt JD, Davies JM. Meeting the need for clear guidelines: Protecting vulnerable adults from improper limitation of medical treatment in institutions. *Law and Inequality* 1986; 4(2):355-378.

Illinois Department of Public Health. *Administrative Code* (Chapter I, Subchapter C), 1979.

Illinois State Medical Society. Guidelines for writing "do not resuscitate" orders. Unpublished, 1984.

Integrate QA: Ethics review to establish standard of care. *Medical Ethics Advisor* 1987; 3:1-4.

Ireland T, Puri VK. No CPR decisions—Documentation and outcome. *Crit Care Med* 1983; 12:315.

Isaacs B, Gunn J, McKechan A, McMillan I, Neville Y. The concept of pre-death. *Lancet* 1971; May 29:1115-1118.

Jay A. The judge ordered me to kill my patient. *Medical Economics* 1987; August 10:120-124.

Johnson SH. State regulation of long-term care: A decade of experience with intermediate sanctions. *Law, Medicine, and Health Care* 1985; 13(4):173-188.

Joint Commission on Accreditation of Hospitals. New and Revised standards approved: Withholding resuscitative services. *JCAH Perspectives* 1987; 7(5/6):5.

Joint Commission on Accreditation of Healthcare Organizations. *Accreditation manual for hospitals.* Chicago: JCAHO, 1988a:90-91.

Joint Commission on Accreditation of Healthcare Organizations. *Long term care standards manual.* Chicago: JCAHO, 1988b:27-29.

Jonas S, Rosenberg SN. Measurement and control of the quality of health care. In Jonas, ed., *Health care delivery in the United States,* 2nd ed., New York: Springer Publishing, 1981.

Jonsen A. A concord in medical ethics. *Ann Intern Med* 1983; 99(2):261-264.

Jost TS. Enforcement of quality nursing home care in the legal system. *Law, Medicine, and Health Care* 1985; 13(4):160-172.

Judicial Council of the American Medical Association. Guidelines for ethics committees in health care facilities. *JAMA* 1985; 253(10):2698-2699.

Kanoti G. Director, Bioethics Department, Cleveland Clinic Foundation, Cleveland, OH, personal communication, October 16, 1987.

Kapp MB. The bioethically informed attorney and the humanization of medicine. *Law, Medicine, and Health Care* 1985; April:82-85.

Kapp MB. Decision-making in critical care: Is the law an impediment or a scapegoat. *Critical Care* 1986; 14(3):247-250.

Kapp MB. *Preventing malpractice in long-term care: Strategies for risk management.* New York: Springer Publishing Company, 1987.

Kapp MB. Personal communication, January, 1988.

Kapp MB, Lo B. Legal perceptions and medical decision making. *Milbank Q* 1986; 64(Suppl. 2):163-202.

Kass LR. Ethical dilemmas in the care of the ill: I. What is the physician's service? JAMA 1980; 244(16):1811–1816.

Kass LR. Ethical dilemmas in the care of the ill: II. What is the patient's good? JAMA 1980; 244(17):1946–1949.

Kass LR. Toward a more natural science: Biology and human affairs. New York: Free Press, 1985.

Katz J. The silent world of doctor and patient. New York: Free Press, 1984.

Knoebbel SB. The effect of cost containment on the practice of cardiology: Predictions. Am J Cardiol 1985; 56:32C–34C.

Koop CE, Grant ER. The small beginnings of euthanasia: Examining the erosion in legal prohibition against mercy killing. Notre Dame J Law, Ethics, Pub Pol 1986; 2(3):585–634.

Kopelman LM, Irons TG, Kopelman AE. Neonatologists judge the "Baby Doe" regulations. N Engl J Med 1988; 318(11):677–683.

Kouwenhoven WB, Jude JR, Knickerbocker GG. Closed-chest cardiac massage. JAMA 1960; 173:1064–1069.

Kyff J, Puri VK, Raheja R, Ireland T. Cardiopulmonary resuscitation in hospitalized patients: Continuing problems of decisionmaking. Crit Care Med 1987; 15(1):41–43.

Lantos JD, Miles SH, Silverstein MD, Stocking CB. Survival after cardiopulmonary resuscitation in babies of very low birth weight. N Engl J Med 1988; 318(2):91–95.

LaPuma J, Schiedermayer DL, Toulmin S, Miles SH, McAtee JA. The standard of care: A case report and ethical analysis. Ann Intern Med 1988a; 108:121–124.

LaPuma J, Silverstein M, Stocking CB, Boland D, Siegler M. DNR orders and life-sustaining therapy: A prospective study in a teaching hospital. Arch Intern Med 1988b; 148 (10): 2193–2198.

Lee MA, Cassel CK. The ethical and legal framework for the decision not to resuscitate. West J Med 1984; 140:117–122.

Levenson SA, List ND, Zaw-Win B. Ethical considerations in critical and terminal illness in the elderly. J Am Geriatr Soc 1981; 19(12):563–567.

Levin DL, Levin NR. DNR: An objectionable form of euthanasia. Univ Cincinnati Law Rev 1980; 49(3):567–579.

Levinson A-J R. Termination of life support systems in the elderly: Ethical issues. J Geriatr Psych 1981; 14(1):71–85.

Levinson DF. Toward full disclosure of referral restrictions and financial incentives by prepaid health plans. N Engl J Med 1987; 317(27):1729–1731.

Levinson W, Shepard MA, Dunn PM, Parker DF. Cardiopulmonary resuscitation in long-term care facilities: A survey of do-not-resuscitate orders in nursing homes. J Am Geriatr Soc 1987; 35(12):1059–1062.

Levy MR, Lambe ME, Shear CL. Do-not-resusciatate orders in a county hospital. West J Med 1984; 140(1):111–113.

Libow LS. The interface of clinical and ethical decisions in the care of the elderly. Mt Sinai J Med 1981; 48(6):480–88.

Lind SE. Transferring the terminally ill. N Engl J Med 1984; 311 (18):1181–1182.

Lipsitz LA, Pluchino FC, Wright S. Biomedical research in the nursing home: Methodological issues and subject recruitment results. *J Am Geriatr Soc* 1987; 35:629-634.

Lipton HL. Do-not-resuscitate decisions in a community hospital: Incidence, implications, outcomes. *JAMA* 1986; 256(9):1164-1169.

Lipton HL. Do-not-resuscitate decisions in a community hospital: Implications for quality care. *QRB* 1987; July:226-31.

Lo B. Behind closed doors: Promises and pitfalls of ethics committees. *N Engl J Med* 1987; 317(1):46-50.

Lo B, Dorbrand L. Guiding the hand that feeds. *N Engl J Med* 1984; 311:402-404.

Lo B, Saika G, Strull W, Thomas E, Showstack J. "Do not resuscitate" decisions: A prospective study at three teaching hospitals. *Arch Intern Med* 1985; 145(June):1115-1117.

Lo B, Steinbrook RL. Deciding whether to resuscitate. *Arch Intern Med* 1983; 143:1561-1563.

Loewy EH. Treatment decisions in the mentally impaired: Limiting but not abandoning treatment. *N Engl J Med* 1987; 317(23):1465-1469.

Longo R, Warren M, Roberts JS. "Do-not-resuscitate" policies in healthcare organizations: Trends and issues. *Health Prog* 1988 (In Press).

Los Angeles County Department of Health Services' Hospitals. Guidelines for "no-code" orders. In President's Commission for the Study of Ethical Problems in Medicine and Biomedical and Behavioral Research, ed. *Deciding to forego life-sustaining Treatment.* Washington, DC: U.S. Government Printing Office, 1983.

Lynn J. The determination of death. *Ann Intern Med* 1983; 99(2):264-266.

Lynn J. Roles and functions of institutional ethics committees: The President's Commission's view. In Cranford and Doudera, eds. *Institutional ethics committees and health care decision making.* Ann Arbor, MI: Health Administration Press, 1984.

Lynn J. Dying and dementia. *JAMA* 1986; 256(16):2244-2245.

Lynn J. Much accomplished but much to be done. *N Jersey Law J* 1987; 120:109.

Lynn J, Childress JF. Must patients always be given food and water? *Hastings Cent Rep* 1983; October:17-21.

Marshall L. Resuscitating the terminally ill. *J Emerg Med Serv* 1985; 10:24-28.

Masterson JS. A survey of VA ethics committees. *VA Practitioner* 1986; June:83-84.

McCormick RA. To save or let die: The dilemma of modern medicine. *JAMA* 1974; 299(2):172-176.

McCormick RA. Freedman on the rights of the voiceless. *J Med Phil* 1978; 3(3):211-221.

McIntyre A. Why the search for the foundations of ethics is so frustrating. *Hastings Cent Rep* 1979; August:16-22.

McPhail A, Moore S, O'Connor J, Woodward C. One hospital's experience with a "do-not-resuscitate" policy. *Can Med Assoc J* 1981; 125:836-837.

Medical Society of the State of Alabama. Do not resuscitate (DNR) guidelines. In President's Commission for the Study of Ethical Problems in Medicine and

Biomedical and Behavioral Research, *Deciding to forego life-sustaining treatment*. Washington, DC: U.S. Government Printing Office, 1983.

Medical Society of the State of New York. Guidelines for hospitals and physicians on "do-not-resuscitate." In President's Commission for the Study of Ethical Problems in Medicine and Biomedical and Behavioral Research. Deciding to forego life-sustaining treatment. Washington, DC: U.S. Government Printing Office, 1983.

Meilander G. The confused, the voiceless, the perverse: Shall we give them food and drink? *Issues in Law and Medicine* 1986; 2(2):133–148.

Meisel A, Grenvik A, Pinkus RL, Snyder JV. Hospital guidelines for deciding about life-sustaining treatment: Dealing with health "limbo." *Crit Care Med* 1986; 14(3):239–246.

Miles SH. Advance directives to limit treatment: The need for portability. *J Am Geriatr Soc* 1987; 14(3):239–246.

Miles SH, Gomez CF, Cassel CK, Zweibel NR. Nursing home policies for withdrawal of life-sustaining therapies. In Cassel CK, Zweibel NR, eds. *Clinics in Geriatrics*. New York: Springer-Verlag, 1988; 4 (3): 681–691.

Miles SH, Cranford R, Schultz AL. The do-not-resuscitate order in a teaching hospital: Considerations and a suggested policy. *Ann Intern Med* 1983; 96(5):660–664.

Miles SH, Crimmins TJ. Orders to limit emergency treatment for an ambulance service in a large metropolitan area. *JAMA* 1985; 254(4):525–527.

Miles SH, Moldow DG. Hospital policies on limiting medical treatment. *Arch Intern Med* 1984; 144:1841–1843.

Miles SH, Moldow DG. Commentary on the Minnesota Medical Associations's do-not-resuscitate guidelines. *Minn Med* 1985; 68:603–605.

Miles SH, Ryden MB. Limited-treatment policies in long-term care facilities. *J Am Geriatr Soc* 1985; 33:707–711.

Minnesota Hospital Association and Biomedical Ethics Committee of Fairview Riverside Hospital. *Limited treatment policies and guidelines: A model for hospitals and nursing homes*. Unpublished, Minneapolis, MN, 1986.

Minnesota Medical Association. Do-not-resuscitate (DNR) guidelines. In President's Commission for the Study of Ethical Problems in Medicine and Biomedical and Behavioral Research. *Deciding to forego life-sustaining treatment*. Washington, DC: U.S. Government Printing Office, 1983.

Minnesota Medical Association Trustees. Control of pre-hospital care at the scene of emergencies. *Minn Med* 1986; 69:86–88.

Mott PD, Barker WH. Hospital and medical care use by nursing home patients: The effect of patient care plans. *J Am Geriatr Soc* 1988; 36:47–53.

Mt. Sinai HOspital, Minneapolis, Minnesota. Living will guidelines. In Cranford and Doudera, eds. *Institutional ethics committees and health care decision making*. Washington, DC: AUPHA Press, 1984.

Mozdzierz GJ, Schlesinger SE. Do-not-resuscitate policies in midwestern hospitals: A five-state survey. *Health Serv Res* 1986; 20(6):949–960.

National Conference Steering Committee. Standards for cardiopulmonary resuscitation (CPR) and emergency cardiac care (ECC). *JAMA* 1974; 227:837–864.

National Conference on Cardiopulmonary Resuscitation (CPR) and Emergency CArdiac Care (ECC). Standards and guidelines for cardiopulmonary resuscitation (CPR) and emergency cardiac care (ECC). *JAMA* 1986; 255(21):2905–2989.

National Institutes of Health: The Clinical Center. Medical administrative policy No. 82-4. Subject: Orders not to attempt cardiac resuscitation. Policy and communications bulletin, medical administrative series (July 12, 1982). In President's Commission for the Study of Ethical Problems in Medicine and Biomedical and Behavioral Research. *Deciding to forego life-sustaining treatment.* Washington, DC: U.S. Government Printing Office, 1983.

Nelson LJ. The law, professional responsibility, and decisions to forego treatment. *QRB* 1986; January:8–15.

Neu SC, Kjellstrand C. Stopping long-term dialysis: An empirical study of withdrawal of life-supporting treatment. *N Engl J Med* 1986; 314:14–20.

New York State Task Force on Life and the Law. *Life-sustaining treatments: Making decisions and appointing a health care agent.* Albany, New York, July, 1987.

Newman RG, Meyer K, Mernick M. The dilemma of "do not resuscitate" orders. *NY State J Med* 1986; January:1–2.

Northwestern Memorial Hospital. Guidelines for do-not-resuscitate orders. In Doudera & Peters, eds. *Legal and ethical aspects of treating critically and terminally ill patients.* Ann Arbor, MI: AUPHA Press, 1982.

Office of Technology Assessment, U.S. Congress. *Life-sustaining technologies and the elderly.* Washington, DC: U.S. Government Printing Office, 1987.

Office of Technology Assessment, U.S. Congress. *Policies and guidelines for making decisions about life-sustaining treatments in health care institutions.* Washington, DC: U.S. Government Printing Office, 1988.

Paris JJ. Comfort measures only for DNR orders. *Conn Med* 1982; 46(4):195–199.

Paris JJ. Withholding or withdrawing nutrition and fluids: What are the real issues? *Health Prog* 1985; December:22–25.

Paris JJ. Personal autonomy over institutional considerations. *N Jersey Law J* 1987; 120:23–24.

Pearlman RA, Jonsen A. The use of quality-of-life considerations in medical decision making. *J Am Geriatr Assoc* 1985; 33(5):344–352.

Pearlman RA, Uhlmann RF. Quality of life in chronic diseases: Perceptions of elderly patients. *J Geront* 1988; 43(2):M25–30.

Pellegrino ED, Thomasma DC. *The philosophical basis of medical practice.* New York: Oxford University Press, 1981.

Perkins HS. Ethics at the end of life. *J Gen Int Med* 1986; 1:170–176.

Peters J, Peraino J. Malpractice in hospitals: Ten theories for direct liability. *Law, Medicine, and Health Care* 1984; 12:254–259.

President's Commission for the Study of Ethical Problems in Medicine and Biomedical and Behavioral Research. *Making health care decisions.* Washington, DC: U.S. Government Printing Office, 1982.

President's Commission for the Study of Ethical Problems in Medicine and Biomedical and Behavioral Research. *Deciding to forego life-sustaining treatment.* Washington, DC: U.S. Government Printing Office, 1983.

Quill TE, Stankaitis JA, Krause CR. The effect of a community hospital resuscitation policy on elderly patients. NY State J Med 1986; 86(12):622-625.

Rabkin MT, Gillerman G, Rice NR. Orders Not To Resuscitate. N Engl J Med 1976; 295(7):364-366.

Rasinski-Gregory D. Associate Chief-of-Staff for Education, Veterans' Administration Medical Center, Long Beach, CA, personal communication, October 1987 and February 1988.

Read WA. Hospital's role in resuscitation decisions. Chicago: Hospital Research and Education Trust, 1983.

Reagan MD. Physicians as gatekeepers: A complex challenge. N Engl J Med 1987; 317(27):1731-1734.

Reuben DJ. Learning diagnostic restraint. N Engl J Med 1984; 310(9):591-593.

Roberts JS. Reviewing the quality of care: Priorities for improvement. Health Care Financing Review 1987; Supp:69-74.

Rosner F. Hospital medical ethics committees: A review of their development. JAMA 1985; 253(18):2693-2697.

Ross JW, Pugh D. Limited cardiopulmonary resuscitation; The ethics of partial codes. QRB 1988; January:4-8.

Rouse F, Cohen E. Letter to the editor. JAMA 1987; 258:2696-97.

Ruark JE, Raffin TA. Initiating and withdrawing life support. N Engl J Med 1988; 318(1):25-30.

Rush JP, Chambers LW, Keddy W. A study to identify who is the responsible physician for each patient in a teaching hospital. QRB 1986; December:426-430.

Rutstein DD. Measuring the quality of medical care: A clinical method. N Engl J Med 1976; 294:582-589.

Ryder CF. Terminal care: Issues and alternatives. Pub Health Rep 1977; 92(1):20-29.

Saunders C. St. Christopher's Hospice. London: St. Christopher's Hospice, 1977.

Schneiderman LJ, Arras JD. Counseling patients to counsel physicians on future care in the event of patient incompetence. Ann Intern Med 1985; 102:693-698.

Schneiderman LJ, Spragg RG. Ethical decisions in discontinuing mechanical ventilation. N Engl J Med 1988; 318(15):984-988.

Schwartz DA, Reilly P. The choice not to be resuscitated. J Am Geriatr Soc 1986; 34(11):807-811.

Scitovsky AA, Capron AM. Medical care at the end of life: The interaction of economics and ethics. Ann Rev Public Health 1986; 7:59-75.

Scott RPF. Cardiopulmonary resuscitation in a teaching hospital. Anaesthesia 1981; 36:526-530.

Sherlock R, Dingus CM. Families and the gravely ill: Roles, rules, and rights. J Am Geriatr Soc 1985; 33(2):121-24.

Siegler M. Searching For moral certainty in medicine: A proposal for a new model of the doctor-patient encounter. Bull NY Acad Med 1981; 57:56-69.

Siegler M, Weisbard AJ. Against the emerging stream: Should fluids and nutritional support be discontinued. Arch Intern Med 1985; 145:129-31.

Smith DG, Wigton RS. Modeling decisions to use tube feeding in seriously ill patients. Arch Intern Med 1987; 147:1242-45.

Society for the Right to Die. *Handbook of living will legislation.* New York: Society for the Right to Die, 1987.

Somerville Hospital Somerville MA. Guidelines: Orders not-to-resuscitate. In President's Commission for the Study of Ethical Problems in Medicine and Biomedical and Behavioral Research. *Deciding to forego life-sustaining treatment.* Washington, DC: U.S. Government Printing Office, 1983,

Southwick A. The hospital as an institution—Expanding responsibilities change its relationship with the staff physician. *Cal West L Rev* 1973; *9*(3):429–445.

Spencer SS. "Code" or "no code": A nonlegal opinion. *N Engl J Med* 1979; *300*(3):138–140.

Spudis EV, Lambeth WA, Simmons P. Determination of "code status" in North Carolina: Still a delicate process. *NC Med J* 1983; *44*(12):785–788.

St. Joseph's Hospital, Mt. Clemens, MI. Guidelines for withholding cardio-pulmonary resuscitation (code blue). In Cranford and Doudera, eds. *Institutional ethics committees and health care decision making,* Ann Arbor, MI: Health Administration Press, 1984a.

St. Joseph's Hospital, Orange, CA. Guidelines for "DNR/No-Code: orders. In Cranford and Doudera, eds. *Institutional ethics committees and health care decision making,* Ann Arbor, MI: Health Administration Press, 1984b.

St. Joseph's Hospital, Mt. Clemens, MI. Guidelines for irreversible terminal illness. In Cranford and Doudera, eds. *Institutional ethics committees and health care decision making,* Ann Arbor, MI: Health Administration Press, 1984c.

St. Joseph's Hospital, Mt. Clemens, MI. Guidelines in irreversible coma. In Cranford and Doudera, eds. *Institutional ethics committees and health care decision making,* Ann Arbor, MI: Health Administration Press, 1984d.

St. Joseph's Hospital, Orange, CA. Guidelines for health professionals in dealing with ethical dilemmas. In Cranford and Doudera, eds. *Institutional ethics committees and health care decision making,* Ann Arbor, MI: Health Administration Press, 1984e.

Starr P. *The social transformation of American medicine.* New York: Nasic Books, 1982.

State of Minnesota. *Patients' and residents' bill of rights.* Unpublished, 1974.

Steinbrook R, Lo B. Artificial feeding: Solid ground, not a slippery slope. *N Engl J Med* 1988; *318*(5):286–290.

Steinbrook RL, Lo B, Moulton J. Preferences of homosexual men with AIDS for life-sustaining treatment. *N Engl J Med* 1986; *314*(7):457–460.

Stephens RL. Do not resuscitate orders: Ensuring patient participation. *JAMA* 1986; *255*(2):224–240.

Stevens MB. Withholding resuscitation. *Am Fam Pract* 1986; *33*(1):207–212.

Swenson E, Matsuura J, Martinson IM. Effects of resuscitation for patients with metastatic cancers and chronic heart disease. *Nurs Res* 1979; *28*(3):151–153.

Takken TA. Mercy-killing in the Netherlands and California. *BioLaw* 1987; *2*(6):1–6.

Task Force on Supportive Care. The supportive care plan—Its meaning and application: Recommendations and guidelines. *Law, Medicine, and Health Care* 1984; *12*(3):97–102.

Thomasma DC. Hospital ethics committees and hospital policy. *QRB* 1985; July:204–209.

Thomson CJH. Treatment of incompetent terminally ill patients: Reflections on the American experience. *Med J Australia* 1982; March 20:246–247.

Tomlinson T, Brody H. Ethics and communication in do-not-resusciatate orders. *N Engl J Med* 1988; *318*(1):43–46.

Toulmin S. The tyranny of principles. *Hastings Cent Rep* 1981; December:31–39.

Uddo BJ. The withdrawal or refusal of food and hydration. *Issues in Law and Medicine* 1986; *2*(1):39–59.

Uhlmann RF, Cassel CK, McDonald WJ. Some treatment-withholding implications of no-code orders in an academic hospital. *Crit Care Med* 1984; *12*(10):879–881.

Uhlmann RF, Clark H, Pearlman RA, Downs JCM, Addison JH, Haininh RG. Medical management decisions in nursing home patients: Principles and policy recommendations. *Ann Intern Med* 1987; *106*(6):879–885.

Uhlmann RF, McDonald WJ, Inui TS. Epidemiology of no-code orders in an academic hospital. *West J Med* 1984; *140*(1):114–166.

University Hospitals of Cleveland. *Limiting life-sustaining treatment.* Unpublished, Cleveland, OH, 1987.

University of Wisconsin Hospital and Clinics. Guidelines regarding decisions to give, withhold, or terminate care. In President's Commission for the Study of Ethical Problems in Medicine and Biomedical and Behavioral Research, *Deciding to forego life-sustaining treatment.* Washington, DC: U.S. Government Printing Office, 1983.

Van Eys J, Bowen JM, Alt J. Creating a code of ethics: Report of the University of Texas System Cancer Center, M.D. Anderson Hospital and Tumor Institute. CA: *Cancer Advisor* 1986; *36*:115–19.

Van Scoy-Mosher M. An oncologist's case for no-code orders. In Doudera & Peters, eds. *Legal and ethical aspects of treating critically and terminally ill patients.* Ann Arbor, MI: AUHPA Press, 1982.

Veatch RM. Choosing not to prolong dying. *Medical Dimensions* 1972; December:8–10.

Veatch RM. *Case studies in medical ethics.* Cambridge, MA: Harvard University Press, 1977.

Veatch RM. An ethical framework for terminal care decisions: A new classification of patients. *J Am Geriatr Soc* 1984; *32*(9):665–69.

Veatch RM. Deciding against resuscitation: Encouraging signs and potential dangers. *JAMA* 1985; *253*(1):77–78.

Veath RM, Fry ST. *Case studies in nursing ethics.* Philadelphia: J.B. Lippincott, 1987.

Veterans Administration. *Guidelines for "do not resuscitate" (DNR) protocols within the VA* (Circular 10-84-179). 1984; October 16 (abstract).

Volicer L. Need for hospice approach to treatment of patients with advanced progressive dementia. *J Am Geriatr Soc* 1986; *34*(9):655–658.

Volicer L, Rheaume Y, Brown J, Fabizewski K, Brady R. Hospice approach to the treatment of patients with advanced dementia of the Alzheimer type. *JAMA* 1986; *256*(16):2210–2213.

Wagner A. Cardiopulmonary resuscitation in the aged: A prospective study. *N Engl J Med* 1984; *310*:1129.

Wanzer SH, Adelstein SJ, Cranford RE, Federman DD, Hook E, Moertel CG, Safar P, Stone A, Taussig HB, Van Eys J. The physicians's responsibility to hopelessly ill patients. *N Engl J Med* 1984; *310*(15):955-959.

Watts DT, Cassel CK. Extraordinary nutritional support: A case study and ethical analysis. *J Am Geriatr Soc* 1984; *32*(3):237-242.

Wetle T. Death as a care option: Withholding treatment from elderly patients. Unpublished, 1984.

Wetle T. Ethical issues in long-term care of the aged. *J Geriatr Psych* 1985; *18*:63-73.

Winkenwerder W. Ethical dilemmas for house staff physicians: The care of critically ill and dying patients. *JAMA* 1985; *254*(24):3454-3457.

Witte KL. Variables presesnt in patients who are either resuscitated or not resuscitated in a medical intensive care unit. *Heart and Lung* 1984; *13*(2):159-163.

Wolf SM. Ethics committees in the courts. *Hastings Cent Rep* 1986; *16*(3):12-15.

Wolff ML, Smolen S, Ferrara L. Treatment decisions in a skilled nursing facility: Discordance with nurses preferences. *J Am Geriatr Soc* 1985; *33*:440-444.

Yarrows SA. Options for care (letter). *Ann Intern Med* 1987; *107*(3):433.

Younger SJ. Do-not-resuscitate orders: No longer secret, but still a problem. *Hastings Cent Rep* 1987; *17*(1):24-33.

Younger SJ, Coulton C, Juknialis BW, Jackson DL. Patients' attitudes toward hospital ethics committees. *Law, Medicine, and Health Care* 1984; February:21-25.

Younger SJ, Lewandowski W, McClish DK, Jaknialis BW, Coulton C, Bartlett ET. Do not resuscitate rders: Incidence and implications in a medical intensive care unit. *JAMA* 1985; *253*(1):54-57.

Zimmerman JE, Knaus WA, Sharpe SM, Anderson AS, Draper EA, Wagner DP. The use and implications of do not resuscitate orders in intensive care units. *JAMA* 1986; *255*(3):351-156.

Appendices

APPENDIX I

Sample Health Care Facility Protocols

GUIDELINES FOR DO-NOT-RESUSCITATE ORDERS*

I. Summary

The Medical Executive Committee has adopted guidelines for the entry of orders not to resuscitate. If questions arise which are not answered by the Guidelines, the Administrator on call should be consulted. The Committee's recommendations are described in full in the following Guidelines.

A. MEDICAL RECORD   Orders not to resuscitate (DNR) should be entered in the patient's record with full documentation by the responsible physician as to the patient's prognosis and the patient's concurrence (competent patients) or family's concurrence (incompetent patients).

B. CHIEF OF SERVICE   The Chief of Service (or his designee) must concur in the appropriateness of a DNR order on incompetent patients. This second opinion should be entered in the patient's record.

The Chief of Service (or his designee) must be notified promptly of DNR orders on competent patients.

C.   DAILY REVIEW   All DNR orders should be reviewed daily.

D.   COMPETENT PATIENTS   Competent patients must give their informed consent to a DNR order. If, however, it is the responsible physician's opinion that a full discussion of whether CPR should be initiated would be harmful to the patient, this conclusion and its rationale should be documented. If the physician and the Chief of Service deem a DNR order appropriate, and the patient's family concurs, the order may be written.

E.   INCOMPETENT PATIENTS   The assessment of incompetence should be documented, together with the documentation of patient's medical condition and prognosis and the concurrence of the Chief of Service or his designee.

If the patient's available family agrees that a DNR order is appropriate, the order may be written.

If there are no available family members, the responsible physician may enter an order with the written concurrence of the Chief of Service.

F.   JUDICIAL APPROVAL REQUIRED   Judicial approval should be obtained before entering a DNR order if:

1.   Patient's family does not agree to a DNR order.

2.   There is uncertainly or disagreement about a patient's prognosis or mental status.

The Administrator on call must be contacted on any case which warrants judicial review.

II. Guidelines: Orders Not To Resuscitate

In certain circumstances it becomes appropriate to issue a "Do-Not-Resuscitate" (DNR) order and to enter this order in a patient's medical record. In all cases, the procedures and documentation described below should be carried out. Observe that in certain cases the Hospital Administrator on call must be contacted to assess the necessity of prior judicial approval. In all cases the Chief of Service should be kept informed as specifically listed below.

The following procedural guidelines have been adopted by the Medical Executive Committee of the Beth Israel Hospital to promote thorough decision making, and to ensure accurate and adequate record keeping and the clear communication of all such decisions. When individual patient decisions present questions which are not answered by these guidelines, or when judicial approval may be required, nursing and medical staff should contact the Hospital administration through the Administrator-on-call who is available 24 hours a day.

A. THE COMPETENT PATIENT A competent patient, for the purpose of these guidelines, is an adult (18 or over, or an emancipated minor) patient who is conscious, able to understand the nature and severity of his or her illness and the relative risks and alternatives, and able to make informed and deliberate choices about the treatment of the illness.

The competent patient may request the entry of a DNR order at any time without prior judicial approval. The attending physician must then consult with the patient to insure that the patient understands his or her illness and the probable consequences of refusing resuscitation treatment, that is, that the decision represents the informed choice of a competent patient. The patient's mental condition should be documented in the medical record. If there is any question about the patient's competence, a consultation should be obtained from the psychiatry service.

The execution of a "living will," if any, should be considered by the staff, but it is neither essential nor sufficient documentation of a decision to order the entry of a DNR order.

In this circumstance, approval of the next-of-kin is not required, and their refusal of such approval is not sufficient to overrule the informed decision of a competent patient. Nevertheless, the patient's family should be informed of the patient's decision and of the Hospital's intention to abide by that decision.

In all instances where a competent patient requests entry of a DNR order, the Chief of Service or his designate must be informed promptly that such orders have been written, even though the Chief of Service cannot deny such a request from a competent patient.

If in the opinion of the attending physician the competent patient might be harmed by a full discussion of whether resuscitation would be appropriate in the event of an arrest, the competent patient should be spared the discussion; therefore if the physician and the Chief of Service deem a DNR order appropriate and the family members are in agreement that the discussion might harm the patient and that resuscitation is not appropriate, the DNR order may be entered by the physician. In such cases, the physician shall follow the procedures described below for orders on incompetent patients.

B. THE INCOMPETENT PATIENT An "incompetent" patient, for the purpose of these guidelines, is a patient who is under 18 (unless an emancipated minor) or who is unable to understand the nature and consequences of his or her illness or is unable to make informed choices about the treatment of the illness.

If an incompetent patient is irreversibly and terminally ill, and death is imminent, DNR orders may be entered without prior judicial approval, if family members concur in this decision. Before entering such an order the attending physician must consult with the patient's family including, at least, the same family members who would be sought out to consent to post-mortem examination. In addition, the attending physician should consult with, and have the concurrence of, the Chief of Service or his designate, before entering such orders. This second opinion as tho the irreversible nature of the patient's illness and his or her moribund condition should be entered in the patient's record as well as the opinion of the first physician.

If the patient has no family who can be contacted, the DNR order may be entered by the responsible physician with the written concurrence of the Chief of Service or his designee.

C. REVIEW   DNR orders for all patients should be reviewed at least daily to determine if they remain consonant with the patient's condition and desires. Therefore, it is most appropriate for the physician to discuss his or her opinion and decision with nursing and house staff from the outset and frequently thereafter.

D. DOCUMENTATION   When a DNR order is decided upon, the order should be entered in the patient's chart along with the justification for the order and notes by all consultants involved. Specific reference should be made to:

1. Summary of a staff discussion regarding the patient's condition.
2. A descriptive statement of patient's competence or incompetence. For the incompetent patient, the record should include a notation of signs or conditions which indicate or constitute his or her inability to understand and make medical decisions on his or her own behalf.
3. A statement of the circumstances of the consent by the patient if the patient is competent including staff discussions with the patient concerning the consequences of the DNR order, and any discussion with the family. For the incompetent patient, note in detail the discussions with the concurrence of all involved family.

E. PRIOR JUDICIAL APPROVAL   If any instance where judicial review is sought, the Administrator on call and the Chief of Service or his designate must be consulted in advance. The decision to seek judicial approval of an order not to resuscitate should be made jointly and the hospital counsel should be consulted prior to initiating contact with the court.

Prior judicial approval should be sought if:

1. an incompetent patient is not suffering from a terminal illness or death is not imminent;
2. family members do not concur in the entry of a DNR order.

F. SUPPORT AND COUNSELING FOR PATIENTS, FAMILIES AND STAFF   Nothing in these procedures should indicate to the medical and nursing staff or to the patient and family an intention to diminish appropriate medical and nursing attention for the patient, whatever his or her situation.

When the incompetent patient is sufficiently alert to appreciate at least some aspects of the care he or she is receiving (the benefit of doubt must always assign to the patient the likelihood of at least partial alertness or receptivity to verbal stimuli), every effort must be made to provide the emotional comfort and reassurance appropriate to the patient's state of consciousness and the condition regardless of the designation of incompetence.

In every case in which DNR orders are issued, the Hospital shall make resources available to the greatest extent practicable to provide counseling and other emotional support as appropriate for the patient's family and for all involved Hospital staff, as well as for the patient.

GUIDELINES ON FOREGOING LIFE-SUSTAINING TREATMENT*

I. Introduction

These Guidelines are applicable to all kinds of life-sustaining treatment and are not limited to decisions to forego cardiopulmonary resuscitation. The term "life-sustaining treatment," as used in the Guidelines, encompasses all health care interventions that have the potential effect of increasing the life-span of the patients. Although the term includes respirators, kidney machines, intravenous fluid, and all the paraphernalia of modern intensive care medicine, it also includes, for instance, physical therapy and special feeding procedures, provided that one of the anticipated effects of the treatment is to prolong the patient's life (see Section III.2.b).

The term "forego" is used to include both stopping a treatment already begun as well as not starting a treatment, because there is no significant ethical distinction between failing to institute new treatment and discontinuing treatment that has already been initiated. A justification that is adequate for not commencing a specific treatment is also sufficient for ceasing that treatment.

II. Statement of General Principles

1. Presumption in Favor of Treatment: It is the policy of PUH to provide high-quality medical care to its patients with the objective of sustaining life and practicing in conformity with traditional and current ethical and medical standards. It is imperative that the professional staff remain committed to this objective by maintaining a presumption in favor of providing treatment to all patients. However, this commitment must recognize the right that patients have in making their own decisions about their health care and in continuing, limiting, declining, or discontinuing treatment, whether life-sustaining or otherwise.

2. Right to Refuse Treatment: As a general rule, all adult patients who do not lack decision-making capacity may decline any treatment or procedure. There is sometimes, however, a reluctance to apply this rule to patients who seek to forego life-sustaining treatment. Thus, the Guidelines are adopted and promulgated to deal specifically with decisions to forego life-sustaining treatment.

3. Decisions to Forego Are Particular to Specific Treatment: A decision to limit, decline, discontinue, or otherwise forego a particular treatment

---

* From: Decisions Regarding Foregoing Life-Sustaining Treatment, Courtesy of Presbyterian-University Hospital of Pittsburgh, Affiliate, Medical and Health Care Division, University of Pittsburgh. As cited in Meisel et al., 1986.

or procedure is specific to that treatment or procedure and does not imply that any other procedures or treatments are to be foregone unless a specific decision is also made with respect to them.

4. Preservation of Patient Dignity: The dignity of the individual must be preserved and necessary measures to assure comfort must be maintained at all times by the provision of appropriate nursing care, hygienic care, comfort care, and analgesics to all patients, including those who have elected to forego a specific life-sustaining therapy.

5. Surrogates and Patients: In these Guidelines, the term "surrogate" decision-maker is defined as specified in the informed consent policy of the hospital. Unless otherwise indicated, the term "patient" includes the surrogate of a patient who lacks decision-making capacity.

6. Physicians' Rights: It is the ethical and legal right of individual physicians to decline to participate in the limitation or withdrawal of therapy. However, no physician may abandon his or her patient until care by another physician has been secured (see Section III.3).

7. Availability of Guidelines to Patients: These Guidelines must be freely available to all patients (and their families), who upon admission to PUH will be given a general explanation of the existence and content of these Guidelines (e.g., through an introductory brochure) and be given the opportunity to name a surrogate decisionmaker in writing. Patients (and their families) will be able to obtain copies of the Guidelines at each patient unit station.

8. Presumption Against Judicial Review: Families and health care professionals should work together to make decisions for patients who lack decision-making capacity. Recourse to the courts should be reserved for the occasions when adjudication is clearly required by state law or when concerned parties have disagreements that they cannot resolve over matters of substantial import (see Section V).

III. General Principles Governing Decision Making

1. Right to Decide and to be Informed: It is the ethical and legal right of each patient who possesses the capacity to make decisions regarding his or her health care to do so. Furthermore, it is the concomitant ethical and legal right of each patient to be provided with adequate information about the diagnostic and therapeutic options (including risks, benefits, nature, and purpose of the options) which are reasonably available.

2. Collaborative Physician-Patient (or Surrogate) Decision Making:

(a) Decision to forego life-sustaining treatment should be made between the patient (or surrogate) and the attending physician after as thorough discussion of therapeutic options as is reasonably possible.

(b)   When a patient is terminally ill and the treatment to be foregone is, in the professional judgment of the attending physician, unlikely to provide the patient with significant benefit, the patient (or surrogate) should be so informed, unless there is evidence that such disclosure would be harmful to the patient.

(c)   A patient (or surrogate) may not compel a physician to provide any treatment which in the professional judgment of that physician is unlikely to provide the patient with significant benefit.

(d)   If the patient (or surrogate) is unwilling to forego such treatment, the treatment may nonetheless be foregone (that is, either stopped or not started) after notice to the patient (or surrogate) that is sufficient to permit transfer of the patient's care to another physician or hospital.

3.   Physicians' Rights: Any physician may decline to participate in the limitation or withdrawal of therapy. In exercising this right, however, the physician must take appropriate steps to transfer the care of the patient to another qualified physician. Such a decision should be made only for reasons of conscience and after serious efforts have been made to dissuade the patient (or the patient's surrogate) from the decision to forego treatment, and after adequate notice has been given to the patient that the physician will have to withdraw from the case.

4.   Informing for Decision Making:

(a)   It is physician's responsibility to provide the patient (or, in the case of a patient who lacks decision-making capacity, the patient's surrogate) with adequate information about therapeutic and diagnostic options so that the patient or surrogate may make an informed decision.

(b)   This information should include the risks, discomforts, side-effects, and financial costs of treatment, the potential benefits of treatment, and the likelihood, if known, that the treatment will realize its intended beneficial effects.

(c)   The physician may, in addition to providing such factual information, also wish to provide advice about treatment.

(d)   The physician should seek to elicit questions from the patient or surrogate, should provide truthful and complete answers to such questions, should attempt to ascertain whether or not the patient or surrogate understands the information and advice provided, and should attempt to enhance understanding when deficient.

(e)   Understanding of options by the patient or surrogate will often increase over time. Therefore, decision making should be treated as a process, rather than an event. In order to provide adequate time to deal with patients before they lose their capacity to decide, the process of informing patients of surrogates should begin at the earliest possible time.

5.   Withholding of Information from Patients (or Surrogates):

(a)   There is a strong presumption that all information needed to make an appropriate decision about health care (including a decision to forego life-sustaining treatment) should be provided to the decision-maker (i.e., the patient or surrogate).

(b)   Information may not be withheld from a patient or surrogate on the ground that its divulgence might cause the patient or surrogate to decline a recommended treatment or to choose a treatment that the physician does not wish to provide. Nor may information be withheld because of the belief that its disclosure would upset the patient or surrogate.

(c)   Only if, in the exercise of professional judgment, the physician believes that disclosure would lead to an immediate and serious threat to the patient's (or surrogate's) health or life, may it be withheld. In such cases, the least restrictive degree of withholding, consistent with the patient's (or surrogate's) well-being, should be practiced, i.e., disclosure of relevant information not presumed to be immediately and seriously harmful should be provided. Since the process of decision making will often take place over a period of time, such information should gradually be given to the patient or surrogate, when possible, so as to minimize the presumed harmful impact.

(d)   Information may also be withheld from a decision-maker who clearly makes known that he or she does not wish to have the information in question, as long as the decision maker has previously been informed of his or her right to have such information.

(e)   When disclosure is purposely limited, the reasons therefore should be documented in the medical record.

6.   Consultation with Family: Patients should be encouraged to discuss foregoing life-sustaining treatment with family members and (where appropriate) close friends. However, a patient's privacy and confidentiality require that his or her wish not to enter into such a decision or not to divulge to family members the patient's decision to forego life-sustaining treatment must be respected.

7.   Ethics and Human Rights Committee Consultation: The attending physician, any member of the health care team, patient, surrogate, or any family member may seek a consultation with representatives of the Ethics and Human Rights Committee at any time. Motive for consultation might include family-staff conflicts between family members, staff-staff conflicts, and unclear moral or legal status of any aspect, including a lack of clarity as to who should act as the patient's surrogate. The goal of such a consultation may include: correcting misunderstandings, helping in the acquisition of needed information, allowing ventilation of emotions and otherwise aiding in the resolution of disputes. In order for patients and surrogates effectively to exercise this prerogative, they must be made aware of the existence and purpose of the Ethics and Human Rights Committee.

IV. Decision Making for Patients Who Lack Decision-Making Capacity

1.   Presumption of Capacity: Decision-Making Capacity in General:

(a)   Patients should be considered, in first instance, to possess the capacity to make health care decisions.

(b)   In the case of conscious and alert patients, the ethical and legal presumption of capacity will govern, unless countervailing evidence arises to call the presumption into question.

(c)   A patient's authority to make his or her own decisions should be overridden only after a clear demonstration of lack of capacity.

(d)   Inquiry into a patient's capacity may be initiated by such conditions as delirium, dementia, depression, mental retardation, psychosis, intoxication, stupor or coma.

(e)   Refusal of specific treatment to which most patients would agree does not mean that the patient lacks decision-making capacity, but may initiate inquiry into the matter of such capacity.

(f)   Furthermore, decision-making incapacity can be a transient condition and can be specific to a particular decision. Therefore, patients who suffer from any of the above conditions may not lack capacity at all times for all purposes, and decision-making capacity may need to be reassessed from time to time.

2.   Rights of Patients Lacking Decision-Making Capacity: Patients who lack decision-making capacity have the same substantive ethical and legal rights as do patients who possess such capacity. The only distinction is that in the case of patients lacking decision-making capacity, health care decisions must be made on their behalf by a surrogate decision-maker. Decisions made on behalf of patients who lack decision-making capacity should, when their wishes are known, replicate the decision that they would have made for themselves had they had the capacity to do so. If the patient has executed a "living will" or any other form of advance directive to a health care provider, this document should serve as strong evidence of the patient's wishes (see Section V).

3.   Formal Assessment of Capacity: The formal assessment of capacity is a process that ordinarily ought to be performed and documented by the attending physician. A psychiatric consultation may be indicated if psychological factors are thought to be compromising capacity. However, a consultation is not required if the attending physician is able to assess capacity without it.

4.   Selection of a Surrogate Decision Maker.

(a)   In the case of a patient who after proper assessment is determined to lack decision-making capacity, a surrogate must be chosen to make decisions on behalf of the patient.

(b) Ordinarily, the surrogate should be a close family member but a friend may occasionally be the best choice.

(c) In the case of a patient who has several concerned and available family members, decisions should be made by consensus of those family members whenever possible.

(d) Where the patient, prior to losing decision-making capacity, has designated a surrogate either formally or informally, the patient's choice must be respected.

(e) If the patient has no family or friends to serve and if the patient so requests while still possessing decision-making capacity, the attending physician or another member of the health care team in consultation with the Ethics and Human Rights Committee, may serve as the patient's surrogate.

(f) In the case of intractable conflict among family members or when there is no appropriate person to serve as a surrogate and the patient has not previously designated a surrogate, the judicial appointment of a surrogate must be sought.

V. Advance Directives

1. Definition: An advance directive is any written document drafted by an individual either while a patient or prior to becoming one, that either (a) gives instructions to a health care professional or provider as to the patient's desires about health care decisions, or (b) designates another person (i.e., surrogate) to make health care decisions on behalf of the patient if the patient is unable to make decisions for himself or herself, or (c) both gives instructions and designates a surrogate. To meet this definition for purposes of these Guidelines, an advance directive need not comply with any particular form or formalities, as long as it is in written form, and it appears to be authentic and unrevoked. It may be handwritten by the patient or at the patient's direction, or it may be typewritten. It may but need not use a preprinted "living will" form or be in the form of a durable power of attorney pursuant to title 20 of Purdon's Pennsylvania Consolidated Statutes Annotated section 5603(h) or section 5604 or a similar statute (including a "Natural Death Act") of the state of which the patient was a resident at the time of the execution of the document. The document need not be witnessed.

2. Effect To Be Given Advance Directive: An advance directive is merely a written manifestation of a patient's wishes concerning health care decision-making. It should, therefore, be accorded the same effect as an oral declaration from a competent patient. That is, should be followed to the extent that it does not request a physician to perform or refrain from performing any act which is criminal, which violates that physician's personal or professional ethical responsibilities, or which violates accepted-standards of professional practice.

3. Weight To Be Given Advance Directive: An advance directive should be accorded a presumption of validity. The fact that it is written in the handwriting of a person other than the patient, for example, should not necessarily invalidate the document, but should be taken into account in determining the weight to be accorded to the directive. Similarly, the fact that the patient who executed the advance directive may have lacked the capacity to make a health care decision at the time the directive was executed may be taken into account in determining the weight to be accorded the directive. In all cases in which an advance directive is to be disregarded, such a decision must be based on more than surmise or speculation as to the circumstances surrounding the execution of the document, and instead should be based on persuasive and credible evidence. A document that is notarized and witnessed, or complies with similar legal formalities for the particular type of document, ought to be disregarded for only the most compelling reasons. However, the failure to notarize or witness a document by itself should not invalidate the document.

4. Probate of an Advance Directive: Ordinarily, there should be no need to seek judicial review of the enforceability of a written advance directive any more than there ought to be routine judicial review of a patient's oral wishes to forego life-sustaining treatment. However, in extraordinary cases— such as where there is conflict between the written advance directive and the wishes of the patient's family, or where there is a substantial doubt as to the authenticity of the advance directive—judicial review should be sought.

5. Procedures for Recording the Advance Directive: A written advance directive must be filed in the appropriate section of the patient's medical record. Further, a notation must be made in the Progress Notes of the existence of the advance directive.

VI. Documentation of Decisions and Entry of Orders

1. Orders: When it has been determined that a particular life-sustaining procedure is to be foregone (i.e., limited, terminated, or withheld, should it become needed) and the above procedures have been followed, the resulting order *must* be written into the patient's medical record by the attending physician or a designate as directed by the attending physician. A verbal or telephone order is not acceptable. Once the order has been entered, it is the responsibility of the attending physician to ensure that the order and its meaning are discussed with appropriate members of the hospital staff (including nursing staff and house staff) so that all involved professionals understand the order and its implications.

2. Progress Notes: At the time an order to limit life-sustaining treatment is written, a companion entry should be made in the progress notes,

which includes at a minimum the following information: (a) diagnosis; (b) prognosis; (c) patient's wishes (when known) or surrogate's wishes (if patient lacks decision-making capacity) and family member's wishes (where known); (d) the recommendations of the treating team and consultants with documentation of their names; (e) a description of the patient's decision-making ability at the time the decision was made and the efforts made to ascertain the patient's capacity.

3.   Acceptable Orders: Each situation is unique, necessitating individual consideration. Detailed orders are usually required in each specific case. However, if detailed orders are not provided, to facilitate communication when therapy is to be limited, one of the following categories should be indicated.

(a)   All but Cardiac Resuscitation—These patients are treated vigorously, including intubation, mechanical ventilation, and measures to prevent cardiac arrest. However, should such a patient develop cardiac arrest in spite of every therapeutic effort, no resuscitative efforts are made and the patient is permitted to die. In those situations where patients are being monitored for arrhythmia control, cardioversion or defibrillation for ventricular tachycardia or fibrillation will be attempted once, unless specified not to by written order. Further, it is understood that a cardiac arrest of an "All But Cardiac Resuscitation" patient occurring unexpectedly, for example, as an iatrogenic complication may be treated with full cardiopulmonary resuscitation. However, this possibility should be discussed with the patient and/or family in advance.

(b)   Limited Therapy—In general, no additional therapy is initiated except for hygienic care and for comfort. Should cardiac arrest occur, no resuscitative efforts are made. Therapy already initiated will be limited by specific written order only. Exceptions may occur—for example, it may be appropriate to initiate certain drug therapy in a patient who had decided in advance against intubation, dialysis, etc.

(c)   Comfort Measures Only—These patients will only receive nursing and hygienic care and medications appropriate to maintain comfort as ordered. Therapy (e.g., administration of narcotics) which is necessary for comfort may be utilized even if it contributes to cardiorespiratory depression. Therapies already initiated will be reviewed by the physician and discontinued if not related to comfort or hygiene.

POLICY FOR LIMITING LIFE-SUSTAINING TREATMENT *

Statement of Purpose

It is the policy of University Hospitals of Cleveland to provide high-quality medical care to its patients with the objective of saving and sustaining life, However, this commitment involves recognition that initiation or continu-ation of treatment may not constitute optimum care when the burdens of such treatment outweigh its benefits to the patient. At these times, the objective is to allow as peaceful a death as possible.

Guidelines and Principles

When such treatment limitation is considered, the following guidelines and principles should apply:

1.   Competent patients must be consulted and have a right to refuse treatment.
2.   The wishes of incompetent adults and legal minors should be given consideration.
3.   Plans to limit treatment must be discussed with the family unless the patient requests otherwise.
4.   Consultation with other health professionals involved with the care of the patient is strongly recommended.
5.   Members of the health care team, particularly physicians and nurses, have the responsibility to provide an appropriate level of assistance to patients in reaching decisions about their care. Such efforts should be carefully coordinated.
6.   Maintaining the dignity and comfort of the patient will receive the highest priority.
7.   Limitation of life-sustaining treatment in no way implies abandon-ment.
8.   There is no morally relevant distinction between withholding and withdrawing life-sustaining treatment when its burdens outweigh its ben-efits to the patient.
9.   If treatment limitation is not documented in the patient's record, as set forth in this policy, the presumption will be that life-sustaining inter-ventions, including cardiopulmonary resuscitation, will be provided.
10.   The ultimate responsibility for implementation of this policy rests with the patient's primary physician.

Source: University Hospitals of Cleveland, © 1987; excerpted from University Hospitals of Cleveland, Cleveland, Ohio, 1987.

The following policy and procedure is intended to implement these guidelines and principles, enhance communication between health professionals, patients and families and to maximize treatment consistency.

Levels of Treatment: Limitation of life-sustaining treatment must be identified with a Level of Treatment order as set forth below when: (1) withholding resuscitation in the event of an arrest, and (2) limiting treatment of other selected life-threatening conditions which might lead to arrest and death.

1. Do Not Resuscitate (DNR)

In the event of a cardiac, pulmonary, or cardiopulmonary arrest, no resuscitative measures will be initiated including mechanical ventilation, endotracheal intubation, chest compression, or the administration of emergency medications or fluids. Defibrillation is allowed. Short of an arrest, patients in this category are candidates for all active treatment measures.

NOTE: If a decision has been made to attempt resuscitation in the event of an arrest, but to limit the resuscitative measures used, e.g., to utilize all resuscitative measures except intubation, this limitation should be specified on the standard physician's order sheet and the rationale detailed in the progress notes.

2. Do Not Resuscitate (DNR) Plus Other Selective Treatment Limitation

In addition to the above DNR other, which only applies in the event of an arrest, treatment of other potentially life-threatening conditions will be limited in the following ways.

(a) Initiation of treatment may be limited in the following ways:

- no defibrillation
- no electrocardioversion
- no vasopressors/inotropic agents
- no intubation
- no mechanical ventilation
- no antiarrhythmic drugs
- no hyperalimentation
- no transfer to an ICU
- no dialysis
- no blood/blood products
- no electrolyte or acid/base corrective measures
- other (specify)

(b) Treatment Limitation may also include orders to *withdraw or discontinue* these or any other interventions.

Procedure

A. Physician Responsibility

1. Document in progress notes, at the time of writing orders, the rationale for the order and the relevant discussions held with the patient and family.
2. Review and complete the Level of Treatment order sheet. Any specific orders related to treatment limitation are to be written on this form.
3. If a decision has been made to attempt resuscitation in the event of an arrest, but to limit the resuscitative measures used, e.g., to utilize all resuscitative measures except intubation, this limitation should be specified on the standard physician's order sheet and the rationale detailed in the progress notes.
4. The Level of Treatment order sheet must be signed by a physician; telephone and verbal orders are not valid. It is preferable that the attending physician sign the order form; if this is not possible, the most senior physician present should sign the order form and the attending physician sign as soon as possible.
5. The Level of Treatment orders should be reviewed as appropriate. A new order sheet must be completed at least once a week when all medical orders are reviewed. If the patient's condition is unstable or the patient is in an intensive care unit, the orders should be reviewed more frequently.
6. An order to discontinue a specific treatment, such as "D/C hyperalimentation," that is not a part of a decision to limit life-sustaining treatment or part of a "Do Not Resuscitate" decision can be written in the usual fashion on the standard "Doctor's Order" form.
7. In order to change or discontinue the orders written on the Levels of Treatment order sheet, the physician must sign the bottom of the order sheet, below the DISCONTINUE order. If the order is being renewed or changed in any way, a new order sheet must be completed.

B. RN Responsibility

1. The nurse acknowledges the order by co-signing the levels of treatment order sheet.
2. Insure that Levels of Treatment order sheet is placed as the first sheet in the Physician Order Sheet section of the patient chart. This page should be the first sheet at all times.
3. The carbon copy of the Levels of Treatment order sheet should be placed as the first sheet in the patient's permanent medical record. It should always be the first sheet.

4. If the order is rescinded or changed, draw a solid red line diagonally from top to bottom of the original and copy of the order sheet; sign name next to line. Remove the copy of the order sheet from the permanent medical record and file with the patient's chart in the section with expired permanent medical record forms. Place the discontinued original order form in the physician's orders section of the chart in chronological order according to the date on which the order was written.

MEDICAL-MANAGEMENT DECISIONS IN NURSING HOME PATIENTS *

Principles and Policy Recommendations

Principle	Practice
Patients have "autonomy," the right to choose health care options, including those at the end of life.	Physicians have the responsibility to elicit patient preferences about treatment decisions, including life-sustaining treatment..
Patients should be provided with adequate information to make informed choices regarding health care option.	Comprehensible information pertaining to rationale, benefits, risks, and alternatives should be provided to allow patient to make informed choices.
Unpleasant information should not be withheld from patients simply because it is unpleasant.	The provision of information, even if unpleasant, allows the patient to make informed choices. Information regarding poor prognosis may also allow the patient to attend to personal matters at the end of life. Such information can be communicated in a humane and compassionate manner.
Although the patient's desires are primary, the physician is not required to follow them if they violate professional ethics of judgment, or if they violate the physician's moral or religious beliefs.	As examples, assisting patients with suicide or treating them with unapproved drugs violates the physician's ethic. Some treatments in terminally ill patients may be medically futile. Limitation of life-sustaining treatment, such as cardiopulmonary resuscitation, may violate the physician's moral or religious beliefs.

* Reproduced, with permission, from Uhlmann et al. Medical management decisions in nursing home patients: Principles and policy recommendations. *Annals of Internal Medicine* 1987; 106:879-885 .

When patients and physicians irrevocably disagree on treatment options, patients may obtain another physician and physicians may withdraw from the patient's care.

Either the patient or the physician may terminate the patient physician relationship. The physician is responsible for the patient's care until another physician has assumed the patient's care.

The preeminence of the patient's choice does not preclude physicians from sharing with the patient a personal judgment about treatment options.

The physician may share his judgment with the patient, but alternatives should also be made apparent. Statements such as "You have no choice" and "You must . . ." are inappropriate.

Advance care directives in the form of "instruction" (living wills) or "proxy" (durable power of attorney) carry moral authority and are helpful guides to caregivers, should patients become unable to communicate their treatment preferences.

Physicians and other caregivers should make advance directives available to nursing home patients early in their institutionalization, when they are maximally competent to make choices. Advance directives are legal, under specific circumstances, in most states. Although living wills refer only to "terminal" conditions, they may be legally enforceable for other conditions.

Patients lacking full decision-making capacity should be consulted to the degree feasible.

Although a patient's memory may be impaired, he or she may understand the ramifications of certain decisions. In these situations, patients' preferences deserve preeminence.

When the patient is not capable of choosing a course of action and does not have an advance directive, the physician should seek to discover the patient's preferences.

Often patients have previously declared to family, friends, or caregivers how they would choose to care for themselves at the end of their lives. If the patient is no longer competent, his or her previous desires should be respected if they can be discovered.

When a patient's desires cannot be discovered, a substituted judgment or determination of best interest should be made.

Some patients who are incapable of decision making have never been capable (such as the congenitally mentally retarded) or were capable at one time but never made their wishes known. For these persons, family (especially spouses) or, if available, existing legal guardians are preferred surrogates. They should provide substituted judgment, that is, seek to choose as the patient would have chosen. If the surrogate is uncertain as to what the patient's preference would have been, they should act according to their interpretation of what would have been the patient's best interest.

In the absence of these preferred decision-making surrogates, a surrogate must, nevertheless, be sought to represent the patient.

Several options for alternative surrogate decision making exist. These options include, but are not limited to, legal guardians, ethics committees, and physicians. Although physicians may have a longstanding relationship with the patient, they may also be heavily invested in the patient's medical outcome. From this perspective, guardians and ethics committees may provide a more balanced perspective for the patient and are preferable surrogates. The physician, however, may function as surrogate if designated by the patient.

When decisions to limit treatment are based on substituted judgments or determinations of best interest, consensus among involved parties is preferable.

Irrevocable differences may be resolved by third parties, such as institutional ethics committees or the courts.

When in doubt about the appropriate course of action, the physician should presume in favor of life.

If patients' desires are not known or their prognosis is unclear, the physician should act to support life.

The physician's desire to sustain the patient's life can conflict with two venerable values in medicine, the relief of suffering and the avoidance of harm.

When further intervention has only the prospect of prolonging the dying process, it may be preferable to limit life-sustaining treatment if this enhances patient comfort.

For patients who are in a chronic vegetative state, it is morally justifiable to limit life-sustaining treatment, allowing the patient to die.

Nutrition and hydration provided by vein or gastric tube and treatment for life-threatening intercurrent illness may be withheld from such patients.

No-code status never means withdrawing personal attention from the patient or limiting attention to the relief of suffering.

Continuation of care and support must be explicitly expressed to the patient and other caregivers and documented in the medical record. Orders may direct action for the relief of pain, thirst, dyspnea, anxiety, and other discomforts, and may take priority over correcting physiologic conditions in the dying patient. In addition, vigorous treatment of potentially reversible superimposed conditions may be appropriate.

Resuscitation status of nursing home patients should be determined prospectively, defined in terms of specific interventions, and communicated to caregivers.

Patient's resuscitation preferences can usually be determined on admission and made readily identifiable in the medical record. Decisionmaking at the time of cardiac arrest is a suboptimal standard of care.

As the patient's advocate, it is inappropriate for the physician to deny treatment on the basis of cost or social allocation priorities.

Withholding costly or scarce medical resources should be based on explicit normative standards such as laws, regulations, or institutional policies and not on physician's personal values.

APPENDIX **II**
Sample Advance Directives

A LIVING WILL*

TO MY FAMILY, MY PHYSICIAN, MY LAWYER, AND ALL OTH-
ERS WHOM IT MAY CONCERN:

Death is as much as a reality as birth, growth, maturity and old age—it is
the one certainty of life. If the time comes when I can no longer take part
in decisions for my own future, let this statement stand as an expression of
my wishes and directions, while I am still of sound mind.

If at such a time the situation should arise in which there is no reasonable
expectation of my recovery from extreme physical or mental disability, I
direct that I be allowed to die and not be kept alive by medications, artificial
means or "heroic measures." I do, however, ask that medication be merci-
fully administered to me to alleviate suffering even though this may shorten
my remaining life.

This statement is made after careful consideration and is in accordance
with my strong convictions and beliefs. I want the wishes and directions
here expressed carried out to the extent permitted by law. Insofar as they

* Excerpted, with permission, from Concern for Dying, Room 831, 250 West 57th Street, New
York, NY 10107. 1987.

126

are not legally enforceable, I hope that those to whom this Will is addressed will regard themselves as morally bound by these provisions.

Signed _____

Date _____

Witness _____   Witness _____

Copies of this request have been given to _____,
_____, _____, _____.

Declarants may wish to add specific statements to the Living Will to be inserted in the space provided for that purpose above the signature. Possible additional provisions are suggested below:

1. (a) I appoint _____ to make binding decisions concerning my medical treatment.   OR

   (b) I have discussed my views as to life sustaining measures with the following who understand my wishes.

_____

2. Measures of artificial life support in the face of impending death that are especially abhorrent to me are:

   (a) Electrical or mechanical resuscitation of my heart when it has stopped beating.
   (b) Nasogastric tube feedings when I am paralyzed and no longer able to swallow.
   (c) Mechanical respiration by machine when my brain can no longer sustain my own breathing.
   (d) _____

3. If it does not jeopardize the chance of my recovery to a meaningful and sentient life or impose an undue burden on my family, I would like to live out my last days at home rather than in a hospital.

4.   If any of my tissues are sound and would be of value as transplants to help other people, I freely give my permission for such donation.

To Make Best Use Of Your Living Will:

1.   Sign and date before two witnesses. (This is to ensure that you signed of your own free will and not under any pressure.)

2.   If you have a doctor, give him a copy for your medical file and discuss it with him to make sure he is in agreement. Give copies of those most likely to be concerned "if the time comes when you can no longer take part in decisions for your own future." Enter their names on bottom line of the Living Will. Keep the original nearby, easily and readily available.

3.   Above all, discuss your intentions with those closest to you, NOW.

4.   It is a good idea to look over your Living Will once a year and redate it and initial the new date to make it clear that your wishes are unchanged.

A DURABLE POWER OF ATTORNEY FOR HEALTH CARE

Ilinois Statutory Short Form

(NOTICE: THE PURPOSE OF THIS POWER OF ATTORNEY IS TO GIVE THE PERSON YOU DESIGNATE (YOUR "AGENT") BROAD POWERS TO MAKE HEALTH CARE DECISIONS FOR YOU, INCLUDING POWER TO REQUIRE, CONSENT TO OR WITH-DRAW ANY TYPE OF PERSONAL CARE OR MEDICAL TREAT-MENT FOR ANY PHYSICAL OR MENTAL CONDITION AND TO ADMIT YOU TO OR DISCHARGE YOU FROM ANY HOSPITAL, HOME OR OTHER INSTITUTION. THIS FORM DOES NOT IMPOSE A DUTY ON YOUR AGENT TO EXERCISE GRANTED POWERS; BUT WHEN A POWER IS EXERCISED, YOUR AGENT WILL HAVE TO USE DUE CARE TO ACT FOR YOUR BENEFIT AND IN ACCORDANCE WITH THIS FORM. A COURT CAN TAKE AWAY THE POWERS OF YOUR AGENT IF IT FINDS THE AGENT IS NOT ACTING PROPERLY. YOU MAY NAME SUCCESSOR AGENTS UNDER THIS FORM BUT NOT CO-AGENTS, UNLESS YOU EXPRESSLY LIMIT THE DURATION OF THIS POWER IN THE MANNER PROVIDED BELOW, UNTIL YOU REVOKE THIS POWER OR A COURT ACTING ON YOUR BEHALF TERMINATES IT. YOUR AGENT MAY EXERCISE THE POWERS GIVEN HERE THROUGHOUT YOUR LIFETIME, EVEN AFTER YOU ARE DIS-ABLED. THE POWERS YOU GIVE YOUR AGENT, YOUR RIGHT TO REVOKE THOSE POWERS AND THE PENALTIES FOR VIO-LATING THE LAW ARE EXPLAINED MORE FULLY IN SECTIONS 4-6, 4-9 and 4-10(b) OF THE ILLINOIS "POWERS OF ATTORNEY FOR HEALTH CARE LAW" OF WHICH THIS FORM IS A PART (SEE THE BACK OF THIS FORM). THAT LAW EXPRESSLY PER-MITS THE USE OF ANY DIFFERENT FORM OF POWER OF AT-TORNEY YOU MAY DESIRE. IF THERE IS ANYTHING ABOUT THIS FORM THAT YOU DO NOT UNDERSTAND, YOU SHOULD ASK A LAWYER TO EXPLAIN IT TO YOU.)

POWER OF ATTORNEY made this _____ day of _____, 19 _____

    1. I, _____

_____

_____

as my attorney-in-fact (my "agent") to act for me and in my name (in any way I could act in person) to make any and all decisions for me concerning my personal care, medical treatment, hospitalization and health care and to require, withhold or withdraw any type of medical treatment or procedure, even though my death may ensue. My agent shall have the same access to my medical records that I have, including the right to disclose the contents to others. My agent shall also have full power to make a disposition of any part or all of my body for medical purposes, authorize an autopsy and direct the disposition of my remains.

(THE ABOVE GRANT OF POWER IS INTENDED TO BE AS BROAD AS POSSIBLE SO THAT YOUR AGENT WILL HAVE AU-THORITY TO MAKE ANY DECISION YOU COULD MAKE TO OBTAIN OR TERMINATE ANY TYPE OF HEALTH CARE, IN-CLUDING WITHDRAWAL OF FOOD AND WATER AND OTHER LIFE-SUSTAINING MEASURES, IF YOUR AGENT BELIEVES SUCH ACTION WOULD BE CONSISTENT WITH YOUR INTENT AND DESIRES. IF YOU WISH TO LIMIT THE SCOPE OF YOUR AGENT'S POWERS OR PRESCRIBE SPECIAL RULES OR LIMIT THE POWER TO MAKE AN ANATOMICAL GIFT, AUTHORIZE AUTOPSY OR DISPOSE OF REMAINS, YOU MAY DO SO IN THE FOLLOWING PARAGRAPHS.)

2.   The powers granted above shall not include the following powers or shall be subject to the following rules or limitations (here you may include any specific limitations you deem appropriate, such as: your own definition of life-sustaining measures that d be withheld; a direction to continue food and water in all events; or instructions to refuse any specific types of treatment that are inconsistent with your religious beliefs or unacceptable to you for any other reason, such as blood transfusion, electroconvulsive therapy, amputa-tion, psychosurgery, voluntary admission to a mental institution, etc.):

_____

_____

_____

(THE SUBJECT OF LIFE-SUSTAINING TREATMENT IS OF PAR-TICULAR IMPORTANCE. FOR YOUR CONVENIENCE IN DEAL-ING WITH THAT SUBJECT, SOME GENERAL STATEMENTS CONCERNING THE WITHHOLDING OR REMOVAL OF LIFE-SUSTAINING TREATMENT ARE SET FORTH BELOW. IF YOU

AGREE WITH ONE OF THESE STATEMENTS, YOU MAY INITIAL THAT STATEMENT; BUT DO NOT INITIAL MORE THAN ONE):

I do not want my life prolonged nor do I want life-sustaining treatment to be provided or continued if my agent believes the burdens of the treatment outweigh the expected benefits. I want my agent to consider the relief of suffering, the expense involved and the quality as well as the possible extension of my life in making decisions concerning life-sustaining treatment.

Initialed _____

I want my life to be prolonged and I want life-sustaining treatment to be provided or continued unless I am in a coma which my attending physician believes to be irreversible, in accordance with reasonable medical standards at the time of reference. If and when I have suffered irreversible coma, I want life-sustaining treatment to be withheld or discontinued.

Initialed _____

I want my life to be prolonged to the greatest extent possible without regard to my condition, the chances I have for recovery or the cost of the procedures.

Initialed _____

(THIS POWER OF ATTORNEY MAY BE AMENDED OR REVOKED BY YOU AT ANY TIME AND IN ANY MANNER WHILE YOU HAVE THE CAPACITY TO DO SO. ABSENT AMENDMENT OR REVOCATION, THE AUTHORITY GRANTED IN THIS POWER OF ATTORNEY WILL BECOME EFFECTIVE AT THE TIME THIS POWER IS SIGNED AND WILL CONTINUE UNTIL YOUR DEATH, AND BEYOND IF ANATOMICAL GIFT, AUTOPSY OR DISPOSITION OF REMAINS IS AUTHORIZED, UNLESS A LIMITATION ON THE BEGINNING DATE OR DURATION IS MADE BY INITIALING AND COMPLETING EITHER OR BOTH OF THE FOLLOWING

3. (   ) This power of attorney shall become effective on _____

_____

_____

4. (   )   This power of attorney shall terminate on _____

_____

_____

(IF YOU WISH TO NAME SUCCESSOR AGENTS, INSERT THE NAMES AND ADDRESSES OF SUCH SUCCESSORS IN THE FOLLOWING PARAGRAPH.)

5. If any agent named by me shall die, become legally disabled, resign, refuse to act or be unavailable, I name the following (each to act alone and successively, in the order named) as successors to such agent:

_____

_____

(IF YOU WISH TO NAME A GUARDIAN OF YOUR PERSON IN THE EVENT A COURT DECIDES THAT ONE SHOULD BE APPOINTED, BUT ARE NOT REQUIRED TO, DO SO BY INSERTING THE NAME OF SUCH GUARDIAN IN THE FOLLOWING PARAGRAPH. THE COURT WILL APPOINT THE PERSON NOMINATED BY YOU IF THE COURT FINDS THAT SUCH APPOINTMENT WILL SERVE YOUR BEST INTERESTS AND WELFARE. YOU MAY, BUT ARE NOT REQUIRED TO, NOMINATE AS YOUR GUARDIAN THE SAME PERSON NAMED IN THIS FORM AS YOUR AGENT.)

6. If a guardian is to be appointed, I nominate the following to serve as such guardian _____

_____

7. I am fully informed as to all the contents of this form and understand the full import of this grant of powers to my agent.

Signed _____

(YOU MAY, BUT ARE NOT REQUIRED TO, REQUEST YOUR AGENT AND SUCCESSOR AGENTS TO PROVIDE SPECIMEN SIGNATURES BELOW. IF YOU INCLUDE SPECIMEN SIGNATURES IN THIS POWER OF ATTORNEY, YOU MUST COMPLETE THE CERTIFICATION OPPOSITE THE SIGNATURES OF THE AGENTS.)

Specimen signatures of agent (and successors)

_____

_____

I certify that the signatures of my agent (and successors) are correct.

_____

_____

APPENDIX III

Joint Commission Standards*

On Withholding Resuscitative Services

MA.1.4   The chief executive officer, through the management and administrative staff, provides for the following:

MA.1.4.11   A hospital wide policy on the withholding of resuscitative services from patients.

MA.1.4.11.1   The policy is developed in consultation with the medical staff, nursing staff, and other appropriate bodies and is adopted by the medical staff and approved by the governing body.

MA.1.4.11.2   The policy describes

MA.1.4.11.2.1   the mechanism(s) for reaching decisions about the withholding of resuscitative services from individual patients;

MA.1.4.11.2.2   the mechanism(s) for resolving conflicts in decision making, should they arise; and

---

* Copyright 1988 by the Joint Commission on Accreditation of Healthcare Organizations, Chicago. Reprinted with permission. Similar, but not identical standards, apply to long-term health care facilities and other facilities covered by standards in the consolidated standards manual.

MA.1.4.11.2.3 the roles of physicians and, when applicable, of nursing personnel, other appropriate staff, and family members in the decision to withhold resuscitative services.

MA.1.4.11.3 The policy includes provisions designed to assure that patients' rights are respected when decisions are made to withhold resuscitative services.

MA.1.4.11.4 The policy includes a requirement that appropriate orders be written by the physician primarily responsible for the patient and that documentation be made in the patient's medical record if resuscitative services are to be withheld.

APPENDIX **IV**

Veterans Administration Model for DNR Protocols*

Veterans Administration
Department of Medicine and Surgery
Washington, DC 20420

CIRCULAR 10-84-179

October 16, 1984

TO: Regional Directors; Directors VA Medical Center Activities, Domiciliary, Outpatient Clinics, and Regional Offices with Out-patient Clinics and District Counsels

SUBJ: Guidelines for "Do Not Resuscitate" (DNR) Protocols within the VA

1.   As it has in the past, the Veterans Administration remains committed to the principle of supporting and sustaining life, employing new life-saving or life-supporting techniques and therapeutic measures in so doing. However, medical science has made us realize that in some instances the

* Reprinted, with permission, from the U.S. Veterans Administration, Department of Medicine and Surgery.

implementation of therapeutic decisions and the application of medical technology may not cure a patient's disease or disability or reverse a patient's course. Some patients who suffer from a terminal illness and are incurable may reach a point where application of additional measures would become not only unwanted but medically unsound. In such cases, the physician is seen as not preventing death, but merely deferring the moment of its occurrence. The significant medical problems then are no longer therapeutic, in the strict sense of curing or treating, but rather ones of choice among degrees of treatment, involving decisions relating to control over the moment and mode of dying. In this connection, the responsible physician faces the problem of determining that continued maximal efforts constitute a reasonable attempt at prolonging life or that the patient's illness has reached such a point that further intensive, or extensive, care is in fact merely postponing the moment of death which is otherwise imminent.

2. The basic policy of the Veterans Administration continues to be that of providing the highest quality medical care to its patients and beneficiaries, with the objective of sustaining life and practicing in conformity with the highest ethical and medical standards. It is imperative that our Medical Centers and their professional staffs and personnel remain committed to this purpose. However, this commitment should not be so strong as to overwhelm a dying patient's decisions or undermine his/her well-being or his/her right of self-determination.

3. Therefore, it is appropriate that Medical Districts and/or individual Medical Centers consider for adoption protocols for application within that Medical District/Medical Center, to deal with the issues involved when terminally ill patients request that Do Not Resuscitate (DNR) orders be placed in their medical records and/or that they not be resuscitated in the event of a cardiopulmonary arrest. Even though such a protocol may have been adopted, it will continue to be VA policy that CPR will be administered to every patient who sustains a cardiopulmonary arrest, where medical record does not contain a DNR order that fully complies with the Medical District/Medical Center established policy. However, it is acknowledged that there will be those cases where, in the exercise of sound medical judgment, a licensed physician who knows the patient may appropriately give an instruction not to institute resuscitation at the bedside of a patient who has just experienced an arrest. Such cases would involve patients who were considered terminal, where death was imminent or expected, and where resuscitative efforts would most likely have been fruitless. It may be appropriate to communicate these concerns to physician

responsible for the immediate care of the patient, in the absence of the physician who knows the patient.

4. DNR protocols established by VA Medical Districts/individual Medical Centers should contain certain specific items:

a. An introductory policy statement which sets the tone and delineates specific ethics, legal and medical considerations that may apply;

b. Specific definitions of such terms or phrases as DNR, resuscitation, terminal illness, and imminent death;

c. A patient-classification scheme, to delineate that class of patients to whom the policy applies;

d. A description of the patient's (or patient's surrogate's i.e. legally appointed guardian's or representative's) role, with respect to the competent, the incompetent, and the comatose patient, as well the patient hospitalized within a state which has a "Natural Death" or "Death with Dignity" statute;

e. A description of the family role, where it is relevant;

f. Requirements for consultation, consensus, or committee involvement;

g. Requirements for the DNR order itself and who may write it;

h. Requirements for the accompanying note in the Progress Notes and who may write it;

i. Limits for time duration of the DNR order and provisions for its review;

j. Requirements for other or additional medical care, short of resuscitation; and

k. Requirements for flagging or otherwise highlighting the medical record in such a way as to indicate the entry of a DNR order therein.

5. The following suggestions or recommendations are made with respect to the items listed above:

a. Definitions:

The terminally ill patient may be defined as one whose underlying condition is considered to be medically incurable or untreatable, in terms of currently available technology, and whose death as a result of the natural history of his/her disease process or medical problem is considered imminent, that is, expected to occur during the course of the current hospitalization. In addition, the definition might also apply to those situations where the physician determines that resuscitation would be of no benefit to the patient, because the natural course of the patient's medical condition would result in death imminently, and the institution of resuscitative measures, if successful, would only postpone the moment of death for a brief period of time, that is for matter of a few hours or days.

b.   Patient's Role:

1.   Competent patients: Where the patient is competent and alert, and understands the implications of his/her diagnosis and prognosis, the DNR decision should be reached by the patient after discussion with the physician primarily responsible for his/her care. If the patient requests that a DNR order not be written, or instructs that resuscitative measures should be instituted, no DNR order should be written or considered by the treating team.

The patient should be encouraged to discuss the subject with family members before making this decision. However, there are some situations where a competent, alert patient might for one reason or another elect not to inform family members of this decision nor to seek their concurrence. Under the circumstances, patient privacy and confidentiality require that those wishes be respected and honored and that the family not be informed or involved. However, the patient should still be encouraged in this circumstance to involve the family in the decision.

2.   Incompetent patients: Where the patient is comatose or otherwise incompetent, or incapable of making his/her decision, the decision should be reached after consultation with the patient's surrogate, or in the absence of such an individual, appropriate family member(s) and the physician.

Should the patient's surrogate or family member(s) disagree with the DNR order, no such order will be written. In the event there is question as to the patient's competence, psychiatric consultation should be obtained. Should the responsible physician feel that he/she cannot in good conscience and sound medical judgment comply with the patient's (or patient's surrogate's or family's) wishes regarding resuscitation, that physician should arrange to transfer the patient's care to another physician capable of appropriately and skillfully handling the patient's medical problems, who can so comply.

In situations where an incompetent or comatose patient has no surrogate (legally appointed guardian or representative) or family members, and the treating staff (including the attending physician) feels that a DNR order is appropriate, consultation should be undertaken with the Director/Chief of Staff and the District Counsel for appropriate court order to be obtained, permitting such a DNR order.

c.   States With "Natural Death Laws":

If the patient resides in a state where statute permits a directive to an attending physician regarding "death with dignity," "right to die," "living will," or similar provisions, prior exercise of that statutory right by a patient may be considered as evidence of that patient's wishes regarding DNR orders, prior to the occurrence of coma or incompetence. However, the absence of such a declaration or directive should not be considered as an indication that the patient would not have wanted a DNR order written unless there is evidence of his/her specific wishes in that regard. Where the relevant state statute provides additional requirements to be met regarding diagnosis, prognosis, informing the patient, recordation, witnesses, etc., the requirements of state law should be followed, where they are not inconsistent with the provisions of this circular.

d.   Consultation and Other Physician Involvement:

The individual with specific responsibility for determining the propriety of considering a DNR order in a particular case is the senior attending physician in charge of the patient's care, not a house officer. In this context, the ultimate DNR decision should be reached by the patient after discussion with the senior physician in charge of his/her care (staff or attending physician). Medical decisions regarding the patient's diagnosis or prognosis should be reached by a consensus of the medical-treatment team. In larger hospitals, this will mean the attending or staff physician, involved house staff, and whatever consultants may be involved in the patient's care (oncologists, cardiologists, etc.). In smaller hospitals, where house staff is not involved with the patient's care and consultants of that level are not readily available, the decision should be reached by the patient's attending or staff physician and the Chief of Service/Chief of Staff. In those situations where there may be some doubt concerning the propriety of a DNR order or the accuracy of the patient's diagnosis or prognosis, a medical ethics or prognosis committee or similar body may be convened on an ad hoc basis to help resolve the problem.

e.   Entry of DNR Order:

After it has been determined that a DNR is appropriate in a particular case and the foregoing requirements have been met, the order must be written into the patient's medical record by the attending physician, rather than a house officer or resident. A verbal or telephone order for DNR is not justifiable as sound medical or legal practice. Once the order has been entered, it is the responsibility of the attending physician to ensure that the order and its meaning are discussed with appropriate members of the hospital staff, particularly the nursing staff, so that all involved professionals understand the order and its implications.

f. Accompanying Entry In The Progress Notes:

At the time a DNR order is written, a companion entry should be made in the progress notes, which includes at a minimum the following information: the diagnosis, the prognosis, the patient's wishes (when known), the wishes of patient's surrogate or family member(s), where relevant, and the consensual decisions and recommendations of the treating team and consultants, with documentation of their names. In addition, there should be some reference concerning the patient's competency, where the decision was based on his/her concurrence, and applicable documentation of any "informed consent."

Where the competent patient has requested that his/her family not be involved in or informed of his/her decision, as noted above, the patient's decision and request for confidentiality should be documented in the medical record by a disinterested third party, not a member of the treatment team, e.g., a patient ombudsman or representative, a representative of Medical Administration Service, etc.

g. Review of the Order:

The protocol should specify the process of review for such a DNR order, and how often review should be carried out. Obviously, any time there is a significant change in the patient's medical condition, the order would automatically become void. As in any medical situation, a DNR order may be rescinded at any time by the physician at the specific request of the patient, patient's surrogate, or family member.

h. Related Medical Care:

It is important that all involved understand the fact that a DNR order is compatible with maximal therapeutic efforts short of resuscitation, and that the patient is entitled to receive vigorous support in all other therapeutic modalities, even though a DNR order may have been entered. It may be appropriate then, in these circumstances, to write onto the order sheet those medical efforts which will be maintained to relieve suffering and assure patient comfort, including basic nursing care (body cleanliness, mouth care, positioning); adequate analgesia; suction; intake for comfort, including hydration; and oxygen for comfort. Merely because a DNR order has been entered into a patient's record does not mean that there is justification for ignoring the patient or providing him/her less than hu-manistic care and concern for his/her welfare and comfort.

6. Conclusion:

   DNR protocols can be developed to effectively deal with the trauma and suffering that frequently accompany the circumstances in which such orders are written. These protocols must give fair consideration to the patient's medical needs, the social and psychological needs of the patient's family, the legal rights and responsibilities of physician and patient, the professional needs of hospital administration and staff, and applicable state law (as outlined in paragraph 5c, "States With Natural Death Laws"). With the assistance of all involved, and District Counsels, sound protocols can be developed and implemented. Obviously, no patient shall be considered for a DNR order in anticipation of possible problems such as might occur as the result of unforeseen difficulties during hospitalization or as a result of surgery or in any case where the patient is not terminally ill. Under no circumstances should DNR orders be written where they are in compliance only with a request for "assisted suicide" or voluntary euthanasia. "Do Not Resuscitate" does not mean that the medical staff will take any affirmative steps to "hasten the patient on his/her way." All parties including all levels of providers should try to provide and improve acceptable therapeutic options available to the dying patient.

APPENDIX V
Selected Bioethics Texts and Journals

TEXTS

These works, selected from innumerable candidates, are representative of those that are especially useful for clinicians. Good reviews of current books may be found in the medical and ethics journals.

Beauchamp TL, Childress JF. *Principles of Biomedical Ethics*, 2nd ed. New York & Oxford: Oxford University Press, 1983. A widely used text.

Brody B. *Life and Death Decision Making*. New York: Oxford University Press, 1988. A new text with many case discussions.

Cranford RE, Doudera AE, eds. *Institutional Ethics Committees and Health Care Decision Making*. Ann Arbor, MI: Health Administration Press, 1984. A review of the ethics committees.

Hastings Center, *Guidelines on the Termination of Life-sustaining Treatment and the Care of the Dying*. Briarcliff Manor, NY: Hasings Center, 1987.

Jonsen AR, Siegler M, Winslade WJ. *Clinical Ethics: A Practical Approach to Ethical Decisions in Clinical Medicine*, 2nd ed. New York: Macmillan Press, 1986. A handbook formatted and written for ready clinical use.

Veatch RM. *Case studies in medical ethics*. Cambridge, MA: Harvard University Press, 1977.

Veatch RM, Fry ST. *Case Studies in Nursing Ethics*. Philadelphia, JB Lippincott Co. 1987. A case book from a nursing perspective.

JOURNALS

These bioethics periodicals are written for clinicians, health facility lawyers, and administrators. Publications primarily for academic specialists are not included.

American Journal of Law and Medicine, 765 Commonwealth Avenue, 16th Floor, Boston, MA 02215.
Hastings Center Report, 225 Elm Road, Briarcliff Manor, NY 10510.
Issues in Law and Medicine, P.O. Box 1586, Terre Haute, IN 47808-1586.
Journal of Law, Medicine and Health Care, 765 Commonwealth Avenue, 16th Floor, Boston, MA 02215.
Medical Ethics Advisor, 67 Peachtree Park Road, Atlanta, GA 30309.
Second Opinion: Health, Faith and Ethics, Park Ridge Center, 1875 Dempster St. Suite 175, Park Ridge, IL 60068

Index

A

Abortions, 17, 62
Abuse of patients, 69
Accountability, 15–16, 20–21
  and interfacility transfers, 79–80
  and treatment implementation,
    76–78
Accreditation standards, 21
  complying with, 18
  as evidence for standards of practice,
    20
  requirements on protocol drafting,
    31–32
  sample of, 134–135; see also Joint
    Commission on Accreditation
    of Health Care Organizations
Administrative responsibility
  in protocols, 20, 36–37, 81
  for vulnerable patients, 69–70
Administrators
  in protocol-drafting group, 31–33, 38
  views of protocols 8, 9
Admission conferences, and treatment
  planning, 65
Advance directives, sample copies of,
  126–133
  use in protocols, 115–116, 122; see
    also Durable power of attorney;
    Living wills
Aggressive treatment, as default
  treatment, 75
All But Cardiac Resuscitation, 50; see
  also Do-Not-Resuscitate Protocols
Ambulance service protocols, see
  Emergency Medical Systems
Amending protocols, 81

American College of Emergency
  Physicians, 10–11
American Health Care Association,
  11
American Heart Association, 4
American Hospital Association, 11
  protocol model of, 34
American Medical Association, 11
American Red Cross, 4
Anderson, William (case study), 43–44,
  49, 51, 56, 57, 59, 60, 62, 64, 67,
  70, 72, 75, 76, 78, 79
Antibiotics, elective withholding of,
  6, 56
Arena, F. P., 52 (tab.)
Artificial feeding, xvii, 9, 44, 61
Autonomy, see Patient autonomy

B

Bar Association of San Francisco, 34
Beth Israel Hospital, Boston, xiii,
  105–109
Bill of Rights, see Patient bill of rights
Bioethical principles, see Ethical
  principles
Brain death, 33, 81

C

California, DNR protocols in, xiii
Callahan, D., 55 (tab.)
Cancer research center protocols,
  61
Capitated reimbursements plans,
  19, 72